GENETIC
BREAKDOWN

GENETIC BREAKDOWN

THE TRUTH ABOUT VIOXX, BEXTRA, AND CELEBREX

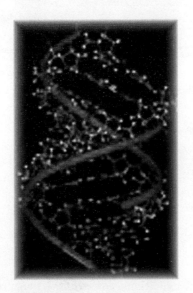

STACEY PRICE BROWN

To order additional copies of this book, contact:
Xlibris Corporation
1-888-795-4274
www.Xlibris.com
Orders@Xlibris.com
42749

CONTENTS

To my husband Ricky and my children Ricky, Eric, and Stacey

I will bless the Lord at all times; His praise shall continually be in my mouth. The righteous cry out, and the Lord hears, and delivers them out of their troubles. Many are the afflictions of the righteous But the Lord delivers him out of them all.

—Psalms 34:1, 17, 19

ACKNOWLEDGMENTS

"We know that no Prophecy of the scripture has ever been a matter of any private interpretation. For no prophecy was ever made by an act of human will, but by men moved by the Holy Spirit spoke from God." (2 Peter 1:20, 21)

Thank you to the several men of God who allowed the Holy Spirit to speak and delivered to me the incredible prophecy. I believe God.

"God is not a man that He should lie, nor a son of man, that He should repent; has He said, and will He not do it?" (Numbers 23:19)

Thank you to my brothers and sisters in Christ, who prayed for me, believed God for me, and encouraged me.

"I can do all things through Christ who strengthens me." (Philippians 4:13)

My wonderful and loving father, James Henry "Speedy" Price, has gone on to be with the Lord. My mother, Claudia Gayle Price, helped me develop my skills and strengths. "Train up a child in the way he should go, and when he is old he will not depart from it." (Proverbs 22:6). My parents gave me a strong foundation in the church. When there where storms in my life, Mother, you prayed and told me everything was going to be all right—and they always were. I love you.

Laus Deo

CHAPTER ONE

What is a Cox-2 Inhibitor: Vioxx/Bextra/Celebrex

Many people suffer from arthritis, which causes an inflammatory response and pain in the joints. An astonishing one in three Americans suffers from this debilitating disease. There are three common types of arthritis—rheumatoid, osteoarthritis, and infectious arthritis—although there are over one hundred different known categories. There is no cure for arthritis. This disease attacks the joints and causes pain and stiffness. The difference between osteo and rheumatoid is that the latter will not only destroy the joints but it will also affect the vocal cords, causing hoarseness. When the disease is finished running its course by systemically destroying the joints and surrounding muscle, it will destroy organs and tissue as well. Osteoarthritis is limited to joint destruction. It will break down cartilage, primarily affecting the hands, feet, and spine. Most people suffering with infectious arthritis already have an existing joint problem that has exacerbated into infectious arthritis.

You've heard the expression, "No pain, no gain." You don't have to have arthritis to reach for an aspirin. Just the pain from working out in the gym or a hard day at the job may require an aspirin. Usually it begins with minor joint pain that is treated with aspirin. When we have a minor ache or pain, we take an aspirin. When we have a headache, we take an aspirin. You can go anywhere in the world, and this is one pharmaceutical that has gained worldwide recognition and deservedly so. The chemical name for aspirin is acetylsalicylic acid, and it has been used for years as an analgesic, which means it will relieve minor aches and pains. It will also reduce fever and inflammation. Aspirin has been the wonder drug and the answer to pain, fever, and inflammation for years.

There is a medical campaign that one children's aspirin a day will reduce the risk of heart attack, and the reason is that the known medical properties of aspirin as an anticoagulant or a blood thinner. Did you ever wonder how taking a baby aspirin daily actually reduces heart attacks? Blood vessels transport blood throughout the body. It is called the cardiovascular system because oxygen is delivered throughout the body through a network of veins and arteries in order for blood to arrive to or from the heart—cardio or heart and vascular or arterial network. Prostaglandins regulate the contraction and relaxation of (a) smooth muscle (heart), (b) the dilation and constriction of blood vessels, and (c) control blood pressure and inflammation. When blood vessels dilate, constrict, or clot, then an enzyme is necessary to make this happen. This enzyme is called thromboxane. There is a process that takes place in the platelets called Thromboxane-A-synthase. It is a process whereby the enzyme thromboxane catalyzes the conversion of prostaglandins (H2) into thromboxane A-2, and the result is a blood clot. When the blood clots, it is because the blood has thickened or coagulated and prevents or slows down the movement of blood through the artery or vein. Blood clots and narrowed arteries are the culprits in heart attacks. Long-term use of aspirin has proven effective in blocking the formation of thromboxane A-2 in platelets. If there is thromboxane A-2 present in the circulating system, then this will lead to thrombosis. *Thrombosis* is the medical term used when there is the formation of a blood clot inside the blood vessel. The presence of too much thromboxane A-2 in the circulatory system will lead to the obstruction of the flow of blood in the circulatory system and, inevitably, to a heart attack. The specific job of aspirin is to prevent blood from clotting by not allowing platelets to produce the "normal" amounts of thromboxane A-2. This is a chemical naturally present in the blood, allowing the blood to clot, in case of injury. **Thromboxane A-2 is produced by another enzyme called cyclooxygenase or Cox-1**. There is no doubt as to the proven benefits of aspirin; however, as with any pharmaceutical, there are side effects. Aspirin has been shown to cause bleeding and ulcers in the gastrointestinal tract.

As we already know, the human body is very complex. After we ingest anything, it goes directly to the stomach, which is considered a hollow organ. This organ contains gastric juices or enzymes, which are prepared to digest and break down food, liquids, or medicine so that the human body can receive benefits. There are digestive enzymes present that break down whatever is in that stomach environment and changes it from large molecules into smaller ones so that they can move on into the smaller intestine. Once there, they can be absorbed by the human body. In order for this to be achieved, the stomach environment contains up to three liters of gastric juices. **Gastric juice is a secretion promoted by the hormone gastrin.** After food is broken down, the molecules called peptides or chemical bonds are then released directly into the bloodstream. Think of the body as a computer. It will detect that there are peptides in the stomach. However, if the body detects that there are too many peptides, then the human computer will continue to send gastric juice and will not turn off until it feels that everything has been broken down. The result is gastrointestinal bleeding. This has been the primary problem of users of aspirin and certain drugs. A drug company attempted to fix the problem by introducing three prescription drugs they felt could selectively block and control the **enzyme** causing the gastric disturbance while relieving inflammation and pain caused by arthritis sufferers.

Aspirin is in the class of nonsteroidal drugs. The name *aspirin* was first used by the German company Bayer, and they held the first trademark in 1899. However, the right to use that trademark was purchased by the U.S. Government and Sterling Drug Company (which became Eastman Kodak and is now Sanofi Aventis Pharmaceutical) even before the patent expired, along with all the patent rights and trademarks in 1917. Today, in many countries, the product is just known by its pharmaceutical name, aspirin, and can be found on the shelves. In some countries, aspirin is still a trademark and can be found under its pharmaceutical name acetylsalicylic acid or ASA. In German language countries, it will be shelved as ASS which stands for acetylsalicysaure; in Spanish or Portuguese language countries, AAS or acido acetilsalicilico; and in French-speaking countries, acide acetylsalicylique or AS.

In 1971 John Robert Vane won the Nobel Prize in Physiology or Medicine for discovering how aspirin works in the human body. He was employed by the Royal College of Surgeons of London, and it wasn't until 1971 that it was understood that **prostaglandins** and **thromboxanes** are the keys to how aspirin controls inflammation and fever and reduces clots in the circulatory system in the human body. He discovered that **cyclooxygenase** or **COX** is an enzyme in the human body, which participates in the production of prostaglandins and thromboxanes. Scientists felt that if they could **selectively block** the chemical messengers in the body that causes inflammation, what a marvelous discovery that would be! Prostaglandin got its name because the scientist who discovered it mistakenly thought it came from the prostate gland. A prostaglandin is, however, technically a **hormone**. In order to understand what a prostaglandin is, we have to understand the function of the hormone in the body.

Hormones

The hormone is a chemical messenger, and its molecules are secreted and released directly into the bloodstream. Hormones can signal the stimulation or inhibition of growth, or they can signal programmed cell death, which is a process called apoptosis. They can activate or inhibit the **immune system** and can also regulate the **life cycle,** which we term puberty, fertility, and, in mature women, menopause. Hormones can also **regulate dysfunction** in these cycles as well.

In 1982, biochemists Bergstrom, Samuelsson, and Vane were jointly awarded a Nobel Prize for their work in Physiology in Medicine, and research on prostaglandins. Then a pharmaceutical company developed a drug based upon their work that they thought could **selectively block** the **COX**-2 enzyme in the body, which causes inflammation. In fact, the pharmaceutical company developed **three drugs,** and the specific function of each drug was to **impede** the production of **prostaglandins.** Prostaglandins, however, were placed strategically in the body by God to mediate communication between cells. Prostaglandins have several functions. One of their functions is to act as a defense when there is pain, inflammation, or trauma to the body. As previously mentioned, their specific function is to regulate the contraction and relaxation of (a) smooth muscle (heart), (b) the dilation and constriction of blood vessels, and (c) control blood pressure and inflammation. There is an area in the brain called the hypothalamus. It links

The Pituitary & Hypothalamus

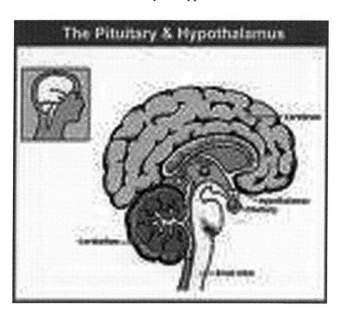

the nervous system to the endocrine system via the pituitary gland, which is known as the **master gland.** The pituitary gland is about the size of a pea and is located at the base of the skull. It secretes **hormones** into the bloodstream, and they in turn can **activate, stimulate, or inhibit your immune system.** A hormone is a chemical messenger signaling instructions from one cell to another. The pituitary controls blood pressure, growth, sex organ functions in men and women, breast milk function, thyroid gland function, metabolism (conversion of food into energy), pregnancy and childbirth, and the regulation of water content in the body.

    Cyclooxygenase or **COX** is an enzyme in the body that **forms prostanoids: prostaglandins, thromboxane,** and **prostacyclin.** They are known as biological mediators. They are called biological mediators because they act to control inflammation, clotting, and allergic reactions in the body. Prostacyclin comes from cells in the blood vessel walls, and its function is to prevent clumping involved in blood clotting.

There are currently three known COX isoenzymes: COX-1, COX-2, and COX-3. Depending upon the tissue, selective inhibition will make a difference in terms of side effects. Prostaglandins can be found in virtually **all** tissues and organs in the body. When there is inflammation in the body, COX-2 levels are increased. Inflammation is the first response of the immune system to infection: redness, heat, tumor, swelling, pain, and dysfunction of the organs. The pharmaceutical company named their drugs **Bextra** or Valdecoxib, **Celebrex** or Celecoxib, and **Vioxx** or Refocoxib: COX-2 selective inhibitors. One purpose that they had in mind was to prevent the gastrointestinal side effects of aspirin. However, reports of heart attack, stroke, hypertension, and renal failure in record number forced the manufacturer to pull the drugs off the market in 2004. The manufacturer claimed that the drug had the capability of separating prostaglandins into good and bad prostaglandins. They claimed that COX-1 could protect the gastrointestinal tract while COX-2 could control inflammation and pain. They claimed they also had test results that could prove the drugs were as effective as ibuprofen, naproxen, diclofenac, and aspirin.

This drug company has made major breakthroughs in medicine and contributions to the world in AIDS research. It is a shame studies proved in clinical trials that the drugs were unsafe in 1999, and they proceeded to distribute them anyway. These drug trials are discussed at length in chapter 32. To date, it has been estimated that there have been between 26,000 to 140,000 heart attacks and sudden deaths and related bodily injuries, depending upon which news report you read.

How the Drugs Work in the Body

In order to understand how COX selective inhibitors work in the body, we have to first understand how drugs work. Since prostaglandins are hormones, the drug specifically goes to work on the endocrine system. Hormones are produced by every organ and tissue in the human body. As previously indicated, **gastrin is a hormone produced by the body and secreted by the stomach.** The endocrine system is a control system of hormones in the human body that secrete chemical messengers instantly because they are circulating via the bloodstream. Hormones act as "messengers" and are programmed to act on specific cells and organs as they flow through the bloodstream. This is due to cell signaling. Cell signaling is a complex matter, as the human body is complex. Cells will respond to signals in their environment. As drugs circulate throughout the bloodstream, drugs act on the cells and produce a chemical reaction. When you ingest any drug, pharmaceutical or otherwise, a process begins to take place as the drug breaks down in your body. The chemicals from these drugs end up in the extracellular fluid of your body, or the ECF, and chemical information or signals are given from there. This information goes directly to the brain, which controls your body and begins to send messages to the rest of your body through your central nervous system. The spinal cord carries these messages to other parts of the body. When a drug is introduced to the body, the general idea is the capacity of that drug to disable or inhibit the chemical translation that is already happening in the body. When we think of the human body as a computer, there is a translation process going on, and the cells are communicating with one another. If there is a drug introduced that interferes and breaks the rules of translation, then the result will be dysfunction or something as serious as death. Translation is part of gene expression in the human body, and the rules of the genetic code cannot be broken; otherwise, it will wreak havoc, as we have seen. There are four phases in translation: activation, initiation, elongation, and termination. This process will be discussed at length in chapter 31.

Cells will communicate with each other through chemical messages or signals. The body can distinguish between the signals. Hormones send out three types of signals: autocrine, which occurs within the cytoplasm of a cell; paracrine signaling, which occurs when there is an inflammatory response in the body; and endocrine signaling, which occurs when chemicals are secreted into the blood and carried directly to the cells.

The drug failed in drug trials, and the result was dysfunction of specific organs: renal (kidney) failure, heart attack, tumors, autoimmune disorders, central nervous system dysfunction, uterus, liver, bladder, skin, stomach, bone, stomach, and gastrointestinal dysfunctions. The drug company also noted that other organs affected also included the heart, lungs, brain, eyes, stomach, spleen, bones, pancreas, liver, intestines, skin, uterus, and bladder. The nervous system, blood, and connective tissue are also parts of the organs affected when drugs circulate in the bloodstream. With that in mind, what could possibly be "**selective**" as to drug inhibition? What's left? The manufacturer produced the drug with the purpose of selectively inhibiting inflammation caused by arthritis without the gastrointestinal side effects.

All cells receive signals from proteins called receptors. Although receptors may be classified into hormones, neurotransmitters, cytokines or growth factors, they are all receptors and are fundamental in the process of cell signaling. Receptors may be found within the cell or on the cell surface. A protein is any chain of amino acids that are converted into enzymes and structural proteins in order for the process to work. Within a cell, there is DNA, and the enzymes cause chemical reactions to allow the DNA to do what it does. Enzymes are proteins that accelerate the chemical reactions the cells need. **Inhibitors** are molecules that decrease the enzyme activity, and some drugs are designed specifically for that purpose. As an inhibitor, its primary purpose is to bind the same receptor in the cell, producing the same effect as the drug.

Hormones are secreted from specific organs to the blood. They are chemical messengers and are involved in causing or preventing cell death, or apoptosis. This process is called signal transduction. The cell converts the signal from the hormone, and a biochemical reaction occurs inside the cell. The process is carried out by an enzyme in reaction to a stimulus. DNA is located inside the cell and

The Endocrine System

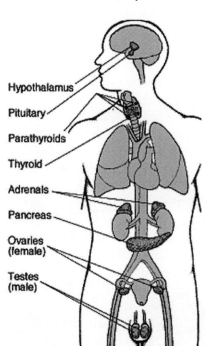

Hypothalamus
Pituitary
Parathyroids
Thyroid
Adrenals
Pancreas
Ovaries
(female)
Testes
(male)

contains what is called a **genetic program**. DNA is actually a **protein program,** and RNA serves as transcription of that program. When the program has been activated and there is a mutation in the transcription of the program, then a **heart attack** will occur, or, in other words, a **genetic breakdown**.

Prostaglandins are lipid mediators and act on the platelet. In **autocrine signaling**, a cell will secrete a chemical messenger called an autocrine agent. In turn, as it circulates through the bloodstream, it can bind to a cell surface receptor from the same cell producing the same chemical signal. **Paracrine signaling** is where the target cell is close to the signal releasing cell, and the signal chemical is broken down too quickly to be released to other parts of the body. This is called the paracrine agent. It affects your response to allergens, scar tissue, the inflammation process, and clotting. The overproduction of paracrine will lead to **cancer**. Prostaglandins are extremely important because they are autocrine and paracrine lipid mediators that act upon the platelet, endothelium, uterine, and mast cells among others, and as such play an extremely important role in the inflammation process. When a cell secretes a chemical messenger called an autocrine agent, it can bind to cell surface receptors on the same cell that produced the signal. An example of this is a mature T cell binding to a peptide, then the T cells can go on and perform their function such as macrophage activation and B cell activation. T cells and B cells are part of the **immune** process. If these cells are inhibited by "**artificial**" sources such as drug-induced selective inhibition, then **autoimmune dysfunction** will result.

The human body can produce all but two of the essential fatty acids it needs, that is why it's called essential fatty acids. These acids are called linolenic acid, or LA, and alpha-linolenic, or LNA. These essential fatty acids can be found in plant oils and fish oils, or omega-3 and omega-6 essential fatty acids. These essential fatty acids produce compounds in the body such as prostaglandins. These prostaglandins are synthesized in the cell from the essential fatty acids and are then released through the prostaglandin transporter on the cell's plasma membrane. Essential fatty acids produce hormonelike substances, which regulate bodily functions such as the immune system, blood clotting, blood pressure, lipid levels, inflammation response, injury, and infection. **Essential fatty acids are also essential fuels for the mechanical and electrical activity of the heart**. During the elimination process of the lawsuits against the drug company, the drug manufacturer automatically eliminated the obese and anyone with a history of heart problems and high cholesterol. High cholesterol is an indicator of your lipid profile or your LDL. It stands to reason that if a COX-inhibiting drug is introduced into the bloodstream that deliberately inhibits the natural function of prostaglandins in the body, the result will be cardiac arrest. Prostaglandins are produced by a process called **cyclooxgenases (COX-1 COX-2)** and terminal prostaglandin synthesis. COX-1 and COX-2 are located in the stomach, blood vessels, and kidneys. Let me put this heart scenario another way. Once the arthritis drug was introduced into the patient's bloodstream, in order for the drug to function, it needed to "inhibit" and regulate prostaglandins for it to effectively work. The human body "creates" prostaglandins by a process called cyclooxgenases, or COX-1 COX-2, which is the natural terminal prostaglandin synthesis in the body. Remember there were a record number of heart attacks and renal failures reported with the use of this drug. This is just one explanation as to why a heart attack could have occurred.

We should be aware of the fact that inflammation has two levels: cellular and exudative. Exudative inflammation involves movement of fluid, such as inflammation of the blood vessels, edema, or swelling. Swelling distends tissue and compresses nerve endings, and the result is pain. The cellular component of inflammation is the movement of white blood cells. White blood cells, or leukocytes, have an extremely important role in inflammation. They filter out capillaries into tissue and act as phagocytes, picking up bacteria and cellular debris. Neutrophils are the first cells to appear in an affected area and are characteristic of inflammation in the early stages. Leukocytes are involved in the initiation and maintenance of inflammation through lymphocytes, which are T cells, B cells, and antibodies. If you were involved in a traumatic accident, mast cells are released. This is the body's response to protect itself by maintaining inflammation. The bone marrow is where blood cells are produced in the body, and it will help defend against infectious disease and foreign materials as part of the immune system.

Autoimmune disease is a condition when an individual's immune system acts **against** his or her own organs and tissues. Allow me to reiterate: COX-2 inhibitors did not allow prostaglandins to function. The production of prostaglandins was inhibited, leading to the domino effect of dysfunction within the body. Scientists felt that once the drug was activated, the inhibitors would be limited to joint inflammation; but they were wrong. Remember, prostaglandins can be found in every cell and tissue in the body. On the surface of the cell, there are transmembrane receptors, which receive signals after the drug has entered the bloodstream. Other than myocardial infarction (heart attack), it has been proven that the presence of COX-1, COX-2, and COX-3 inhibitors has produced a negative effect on various cell types. There are currently nine known receptors of prostaglandins on various cells types.

Nine Receptors of Prostaglandins in the Human Body:

One
GPCR/Immune System/Mast Cells

The first one is called a G-protein-coupled receptor, or GPCR. The GPCR has many functions in the human body. One of its functions is to regulate immune activity and inflammation. GPCRs also regulate the autonomic nervous system transmission: this system is responsible for the heart, blood pressure, heart rate, and digestive processes. Now let's follow the process. We now know that prostaglandins are produced by the human body. It is a natural process called sequential oxidation that will produce all three COX enzymes in the human body. The first is called the sequential oxidation of AA. AA is an abbreviation for arachidonic acid. It is an omega-6 fatty acid, the same acid found in peanut oil. The second naturally occurring sequential oxidation is called DGLA, or gamma-linolenic acid, which is also an omega-6 fatty acid; however, this is one that can also be found in vegetable oil. After the sequential oxidation of AA and DGLA by the body, they become cyclooxygenase or COX-1 and COX-2. COX-1 and COX-2 can be found in the blood vessels, kidneys, and stomach. COX-3, however, or eicosapentaenoic acid (EPA) is an omega-3 fatty acid. This acid is polyunsaturated, and it can also be obtained in breast milk or by eating salmon or fish oil. Prostaglandin levels are increased when there is a natural response to inflammation in the body. EPA has been shown to inhibit platelet aggregation or the formation of blood clots.

GPCRs regulate the **immune system**. The immune system is composed of cells, organs, and tissues, and is arranged in an elaborate communications network designed to protect the body from infection. There are all types of cells and programmed cell death, inflammation, and fever designed by God to protect the body. The body will respond to infection in all sorts of ways we never imagined.

Mast Cells

Prostaglandins act upon mast cells, which are resident cells of connective tissue and are considered part of the immune system. A mast cell contains granules rich in histamine and heparin. As such, they play an active role in wound healing. Mast cells are present in the skin, blood vessels, mucosa of the lungs and digestive tract, and in the mouth and nose. When activated, mast cells release granules and hormonal mediators. These granules are preformed mediators: histamines, mainly heparin, which will act as an anticoagulant, and newly formed lipid mediators, prostaglandins. Histamine dilates blood vessels, making them leaky; and that, in turn, activates the endothelium. This leads to edema, warmth, redness, and the release of other inflammatory cells. This irritates the nerve endings, and the response is itchiness and pain. Mast cells are implicated with autoimmune disorders such as rheumatoid arthritis and multiple sclerosis. Inflammatory cells are in the joints and skin, and mast cells are innate to the immune response and are important in clearing bacteria and viruses.

Two
Uterine Cells

Prostaglandins also act upon uterine cells, which include the major reproductive organs in a woman, and are responsible for uterine malformations. This includes instances in which the uterus becomes thickened: adenomyosis. Other abnormalities may also occur such as fibroid tumors, leiomymata, nabothian cysts, and secretory endometrium. During menses, the endometrium releases prostaglandins and results in some women experiencing painful menses. This is caused by the lining of the uterus contracting, resulting in muscular spasms due to higher levels of prostaglandins, which have been dispatched. The buildup and thickening of the uterine lining and painful aftermath is called endometriosis.

Three
Hollow Organs

Prostaglandins act on vascular smooth muscle cells causing constriction or dilation in nonstriated muscle found within the walls of hollow organs. Hollow organs are defined as blood vessels, heart, uterus, bladder, kidneys, stomach, and the gastrointestinal tract. The contractile function of vascular smooth muscle sets the level of blood pressure as previously discussed. Thousands of Americans have high blood pressure and were eliminated from suing the drug manufacturer as a result of this preexisting condition.

Four
Platelets/Blood Cells

Another receptor is prostaglandin, and they have an effect on platelets or blood cells. Blood cells are produced in the bone marrow, and prostaglandins affect them by causing aggregation or disaggregation—the ability of the blood to clot. Where there is dysfunction, the blood will not clot, and there will be abnormal bleeding. The progenitor cell for platelets is called the megakaryocyte. This large cell sheds cells into the circulation. The circulating life of a platelet is nine to ten days, and then they regenerate in the bone marrow. Prostaglandins are also involved in the function of hormone production and platelet count. A normal platelet count will assist the body in the healing process if you should receive a cut or bruise. When the body is involved in a traumatic accident, normal platelet counts are imperative in achieving clotting factors, the inflammatory response, and the ability of mast cells to respond and to halt bleeding. All these aforementioned bodily functions need to be simultaneously responsive at such a critical time.

Five
Neuron Cells

When we think of the spinal cord, we think of a long column of bones composed of discs, nerves, and cushions. If that column of bone were injured in any way due to activities caused by running, jumping, walking, injury, or disease, then these things begin to affect the other parts of your body. There are things that we take for granted, such as using the bathroom, not feeling pain on a daily basis, or not breathing normally. When prostaglandins begin to act on spinal neurons, they desensitize your ability to fight the pain that you already feel. Neurons are cells that can be found in the brain, spinal cord, and in the nerves and the ganglia of the peripheral nervous system. They transmit electrical signals and are a major class of cells found in the nervous system. There are three different classes of neurons: afferent neurons, efferent neurons, and interneurons. Afferent neurons transmit information from tissues and organs to the central nervous system. Efferent neurons transmit information from the central nervous system to the effector cells, which are lymphocytes engaged in secreting antibodies. Interneurons connect neurons within specific regions of the central nervous system. If you suffer from a spinal cord injury, depending on where and how you are injured, the efferent neuron will transmit signals from the central nervous system to the effector cells, which are also known as motor neurons; and these will affect movement and pain sensation.

Six
Mutations in Gap Junction: Genetic Disorders and Cardiac Disturbance

Prostaglandins have a wide variety of actions including, but not limited to, regulating muscular constriction and mediating inflammation. Molecules and ions that pass between the cells are called a gap junction. Generally the gene coding for gap junctions are classified into one of three groups: A, B, or C. Gap junctions are important in cardiac muscle. For example, the signal to contract will be passed between the gap junctions, allowing the heart to contract in tandem. Gap junctions are present in virtually all tissues of the human body including the skin. Several human genetic disorders have now been associated with mutations in gap junction genes.

Seven
Calcium Movement

Prostaglandins affect calcium movement in the body. Calcium is essential for muscle contraction, oocyte activation, which is a cell that undergoes a process to produce an ovum, building strong bones and teeth, producing clotting factors, regulating heartbeat, nerve pulse transmission, and fluid balance within cells. A deficit can affect bone and tooth formation, and over-retention causes kidney stones.

Eight
Hormone Regulation

Prostaglandins affect hormone regulation. As previously discussed in detail, prostaglandins regulate hormones and control cell growth. The human body is a huge communications network. It is constantly signaling, analyzing, receiving, and converting signals and then acting on these signals in order to function properly. The function of the hormone is to carry the messages that the cells are sending to each other. This is achieved via a "chemical phone," if you will. God, in his infinite wisdom, allowed the body to discriminate, and only the "target" cells will receive the information intended for them. In turn, the cells will respond and give the "target tissue" to receive the message the signal transduction response. The "chemical phone" line is interrupted when a drug is introduced into the bloodstream that affects prostaglandins and will ultimately change the message. The drug manufacturer was well aware of these facts.

Nine
Homeostatic Balance

The final prostaglandin receptor is thromboxane. Thromboxane is named for its role as a vasoconstrictor and creating homeostatic balance in the circulatory system. **Thromboxane, prostaglandin,** and **prostacyclin** are all biological mediators called prostanoids, which are the **pharmaceutical** cyclooxygenase or **COX enzymes.**

All three of these COX enzymes can be pharmacologically inhibited with over-the-counter aspirin and ibuprofen, and have been shown to also inhibit the synthesis of prostaglandins. So it begs the question, were the three drugs medically necessary when over-the-counter aspirin or ibuprofen could do the same job? I know, we are back to gastrointestinal bleeding, but that is a small price to pay compared to sudden cardiac arrest. Alas, back to the drawing board.

Tumorigenisis

Selective inhibition can make the difference in terms of side effects and can have a central role in tumorigenisis. Tumorigenisis is the collection of complex genetic diseases characterized by multiple defects in the homeostatic mechanisms that regulate cell growth, proliferation, and differentiation. When damaged cells survive, or when there is uncontrolled proliferation, the result is a tumor or cancer. This is why cell death is so important and why selective inhibition causes severe side effects.

The Largest Recorded Victory against the Drug Manufacturer

On August 19, 2005, a widow was awarded $253.5 million dollars in punitive damages against a drug manufacturer for the death of her husband after he ingested Vioxx, prescribed by his doctor to relieve arthritis pain. He suffered a fatal heart attack at the age of fifty-nine. Plaintiff's attorney portrayed him as an average worker, a marathon runner, healthy, Joe America—if you will—who was taken away suddenly from the plaintiff and her family after the manufacturer did not disclose the known hidden dangers of the drug. The laws of the state of Texas automatically reduced the verdict to $26.1 million. The drug manufacturer has spent over $1 billion in attorney's fees, vowing not to settle any of the 45,000 claims against it. In an article published in the *New York Times* on August 21, 2007, the plaintiff, at the age of sixty-two, was still waiting to taste the fruit of victory. If it is up to the drug manufacturer, she will still be waiting well into the afterlife. The drug manufacturer would rather line the pockets of high-powered attorneys to the tune of over $1 billion to date than admit that one of the three drugs caused the death of or injured anyone.

In pretrial discovery, the drug manufacturer was successful in dismissing thousands of litigants who were obese, had a history of high cholesterol, smoked, had a history of heart disease, **high blood pressure,** or a combination of these; and all the while, it knew these aforementioned medical conditions had absolutely **nothing** to do with the drug causing death or injury to the heart. Further, the drug manufacturer knew the drugs were responsible for causing a host of other medical conditions that will be discussed at length in this book.

On November 9, 2007, the drug giant finally took a bow and agreed to settle; however, under the terms of the agreement, they specifically would **not** admit causation or fault as one of the enumerated terms of the settlement. In a sudden turn of events, with 26,000 lawsuits remaining, representing over 46,000 plaintiffs, the drug giant agreed to settle and pay $4.85 billion dollars into a settlement fund. The fund was set up to cover federal and state court cases. Regarding the Texas widow and others similarly situated, they may expect to receive recovery as early as August 2008.

Once the individual litigants and potential class action litigants have been pooled, they then may divide the settlement. Four judges have been assigned to coordinate all lawsuits. As previously indicated, legal expenses have exceeded $1 billion, and the drug company has reserved an equal amount to liquidate the settlement fund.

In order to qualify for recovery you first must be a United States citizen, and your case must have been filed on or before November 8, 2007. The litigant must provide physical proof that the victim ingested a minimum of thirty Vioxx pills, and that the pills caused "injury," under the terms of the law, or ischemic stroke.

An ischemic stroke occurs when a blood clot forms in an artery in the brain and blocks the supply of blood. It occurs more frequently in African Americans; however, the risk increases with age. The funds were divided by the company: $4 billion for medical injury claims and $850 million for ischemic stroke claims. The funds are fixed. This means that under enumerated terms of the agreement, this nightmare has finally come to an end for all concerned parties.

CHAPTER TWO

The Beginning

In the beginning God created the heavens and the earth. The water was pure and unpolluted, and the land was pristine. The air was fresh and filled with a symphony of the wonderful smell of flowers, fruit, grass, herbs, and spices that were not masked with the smell of foul pollution. Man lived in harmony with the many creatures of the earth. Life was simple and pure. Some of those animals are extinct because of man's practices. There is a difference between the natural processes of natural selection, which is known as survival of the fittest. However, these processes have been rapidly accelerated because of man's practices from the beginning of time. Man will consume more plants and animals faster than they can reproduce. As such, man has tried to outdo God by genetically altering these processes. We will never see the infamous dodo birds, who were native to an island called Mauritius in the Indian Ocean. Approximately eighty years after they were discovered by the Dutch sailors, they became extinct because the animals they brought to the island destroyed the dodo nests, and the destruction of the forests cut off the dodo's food supply. Man is constantly finding ways to genetically alter the production of food and animal reproduction. Secondly, the introduction of an alien species to a continent will wreak havoc on the ecosystem. History reveals that although early man enjoyed simple pleasures, life was not disease-free. The Bible makes reference to a disease called leprosy, which is a chronic, infectious, granulomatous disease occurring in tropical and subtropical regions. Someone having this disease was declared "unclean" because the disease was highly contagious. The disease is caused by a bacillus. A bacillus is a bacterium that produces ulceration, causes nutritive disturbances, gangrene, and paralysis. Today, it is known as Hansen's disease, and it still affects millions. It is spread by an airborne infection, and all it takes is one drop to infect many. The skin's surface has a loose scurfy scaly appearance. The first sign of illness is loss of feeling in a patch of skin. If left untreated, it leads to blindness, loss of limbs, severe nerve damage, paralysis, and injury to the face, hands, and feet. It is curable with multidrug therapy; however, many children suffer needlessly in Brazil, India, and

Indonesia because of economic hardship. These precious children are our future. We have been aware of bacteria attacking the human body and causing illness since biblical times.

Bacterium exists in a wide variety of forms. There is good bacterium such as penicillin. It is the natural result of a natural set of circumstances set in motion to produce a desired result. There is bad bacterium such as bacillus, as previously discussed; however, this appeared naturally like a fungus or yeast that just got out of hand.

This is leprosy, and despite all our modern medicine, it still exists today.

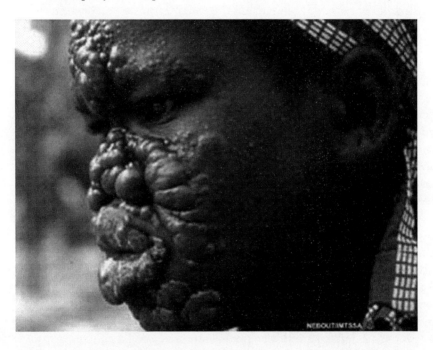

As the population of the world increased, our knowledge increased. As our knowledge increased, so did the need for the use of our natural resources: air, land, water, agriculture, and farm animals. Everything began to grow simultaneously, but we did not notice until it was too late that this growth was a two-edged sword. In less than two centuries, man created an industrial and technological revolution that squandered man's resources. Man ignored the rules and applied shortcuts in spite of warnings and danger signs. Man discovered chemicals and began to combine them. As a result, chemical compounds were introduced into the environment. Man did not take the time to think through a proper disposal process, and, as a result, many of these chemicals were dumped into our water systems; some were allowed to escape into our atmosphere, some were packed into barrels, and others were buried in landfills. The chemicals leaked and harmed the land and affected the streams and rivers. Now in 2007, we are facing an unprecedented drought in the southern United States. With land covering approximately 30 percent of the earth's surface and water the other 70 percent, we would never have imagined water becoming scarce. The plant life and animals depend upon the water and land to survive. To sum it up, man created a toxic, harsh environment that he was not destined to live in. There are over 6.5 million synthetic chemical compounds that did not exist before the chemical revolution, many of which our body cannot identify or cope with. Each year a new compound is discovered. We have a public health crisis because of pollutants in the water. How do we measure the cost of contamination? Is it a coincidence that one in every three women and one in every three men will get some form of cancer in their lifetimes? Today, prostate cancer and Alzheimer's are diseases that are becoming more common among our populace.

Laws were implemented not only to assure that we maintain structure as a society but they were implemented to keep us alive. God gave us laws of social order, which can be found in various places throughout the Bible; the various laws can be found in Leviticus, the Ten Commandments, and Proverbs. If you look closely at the language in our social laws, you will see that they are, in fact, "borrowed" from the Bible. These laws are the foundation upon which our Constitution was created, and they are the very legs upon which society stands on. History tells us that Samuel traveled from year to year "in circuit to Beth'-el, and Gil'gal, and Miz'peh, and judged Israel in all those places." I Samuel 7:16 tells us that Samuel was a judge of the circuit court. This "tradition," found in the Bible, was borrowed or modified somewhat and is being used today. We say things like, "God forbid" (I Samuel 12:23), or a homeboy thinks he is so cool when he says he is going to give somebody a "beat down," phrase found in Judges 9:45. Our traditional census comes from the Bible: so "that I may know the number of my people" (2 Samuel 24:2). The phrase, "In God We Trust," comes from Psalm 55:23, "But Thou, O God . . . I will trust in thee. The phrase appears again in Romans 15:12, "In Him Shall the Gentiles Trust." To the atheists I say, you will not win this argument because you know the United States government is **not** going to reprint all the money.

It is the purpose of dietary laws to keep our bodies from becoming sick and diseased. I recently discovered that the FDA allows the use of the cochineal female beetle as a red dye in our food. The process is to dry out the red female cactus-eating beetle and its eggs, and grind it into a fine powder. I was sickened when I found this out because I am vegetarian and strawberry yogurt is a main part of my diet, not yogurt ala cochineal beetle. I unknowingly was ingesting these disgusting beetles, which also violated my religious beliefs. It is used in varieties of cheddar cheese, dairy products, Smarties candies, marinades, jams, gelatins, processed poultry products, cookies, desserts, sauces, juices, beverages, sausages, pie fillings, and even skin care products, pills, and makeup. The average person unknowingly ingests two drops of carminic acid each year with food or pharmaceutical products; you are not going to win trying to figure out where the bugs are, so bottoms up.

The little white dots all over the cactus are cochineal beetle eggs. They are also used as a dye in clothing, etc.

Cochineal Beetle

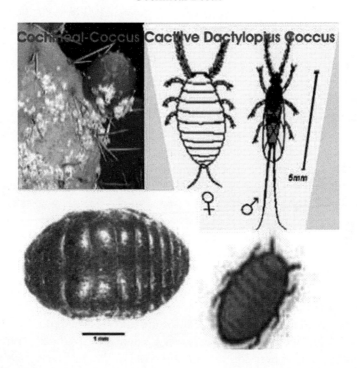

These laws can be found in the Holy Bible: Leviticus chapter 11 and Deuteronomy chapter 19. Yet despite our best efforts, the environment and the denaturing of food has led to the unprecedented spread of disease. God made these bodies, so it makes sense that he would know what would keep us healthy. He also gave us laws to feed the livestock. These laws were violated. Man eats whatever tastes good—from monkey brains to roasted frogs. Those of us without such an exotic diet and have a "regular" or a vegetarian diet are still victim of man's denaturing of this environment. The nitrates found in a hotdog or the edible skins from a piece of fruit because of the pesticides are enough to cause cancer. The soil has been raped with chemicals, and the water needed to grow the vegetables and fruit is toxic. Man chose to chemically alter the genetic structure of our animals by making them produce more eggs or to make their beef tenderer or to mass-produce their feed. They started a process called factory farming, and the cattle were no longer grazing in the fields. They were locked up side by side in stalls no larger than their own bodies, with no fresh air; and they were injected with hormones and other chemicals to fatten them up for market. The farmers noticed that the cattle were not reacting, like dumb animals. They were, in fact, aware of their surroundings and their horrible living conditions and had to be fed large amounts of antibiotics because now their immune systems were responding to the lack of exercise, lack of fresh air, and the stench. The cattle farmers know how to cut costs because their medical bills were sky high because of the use of all the antibiotics and hormones so the cattle, who were by nature herbivores, were fed their ground-up buddies who couldn't handle it as well as euthanized humane society animals, cats and dogs, road kill, and parts of animals that were not fit for human consumption. This whole process is called **rendering**. That's just a nice name for just plain nasty. The result was mad cow disease. The ranchers did the same thing to the sheep, and they began to scrape themselves against the fence and any object they could find and injure themselves. The disease started in the intestines, went straight to the brain, and then death resulted within a year. The disease in sheep is called scrapie, and the disease in humans is called Creutzfeldt-Jacob disease, which is named after the doctors who first described the symptoms. Did we run out of grass and cowboys?

Scientists discovered a protein called a prion (pronounced preeon) that contains no DNA or RNA. They felt that prions will appear in a sick and dying body in response to an illness in both animals and man when the diseased body has engaged in "a grossly improper" diet and unhealthy lifestyle. Prions are a response to the illness in the body and were discovered in 1997 by neurologist Dr. Stanley Prusiner, University of California. He was awarded a Nobel Prize in Physiology and Medicine for his discovery. Scientists have been aware of these protein molecules for over 150 years, but it was Dr. Prusiner who gave it a name. It is an acronym for proteinaceous infectious particles: prion. They are slow acting and inevitably fatal. Scientists have conducted tests, and there is **no way to destroy a prion.** They cannot be frozen, incinerated, or radiated.

I remember as a child in the early 1960s licking the cake pan after my mother made a homemade cake. I remember when my father made a milkshake from raw eggs, vanilla flavoring, sugar, and milk. There was no such thing as Alzheimer's disease when I was growing up. Today, because of feeding practices, the eggs cannot be eaten raw. The world has changed so dramatically since biblical times. It is true medicine and the sciences have advanced dramatically, but it is also true that there are many diseases that exist today that did not exist years ago. That is why the National Organization for Rare Disorders Inc. was founded in 1983. Generally, it is a nonprofit charitable organization dedicated to helping people with rare "orphan" diseases. There are approximately twenty-five million people living in the United States affected by an estimated nine hundred rare medical conditions. This organization is dedicated to the identification, treatment, and cure of rare disorders through education, advocacy, research, and service. Most people that seek out help from NORD usually are affected with one disorder. I believe most rare disorders are the result of genetic predisposition. The rest are the direct result of cellular breakdown caused by the onslaught of these chemical compounds on the human body over time. These diseases are the result of dormant DNA

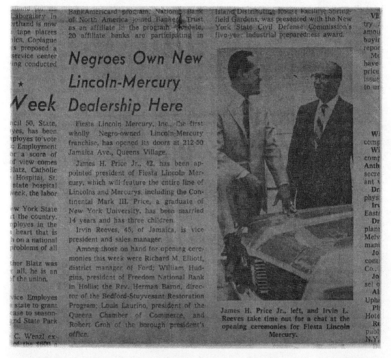

that becomes active after two people, who have no idea this would be the result, procreate. I believe I am the result of a combination of both case scenarios. What are the chances that one person would be affected with over nine rare disorders, one of which is not listed in their database? That one rare disease makes me one of 214 in the world. I guess I would be called a medical anomaly. It is a miracle, and by the grace of God that I am still alive. I believe that it is the grace of God that keeps me going. It is why I decided to write this book—to educate and advocate. What I am experiencing is a genetic breakdown—both hereditary and drug induced. I ingested Vioxx over a six-month period for osteoarthritis, and then my pain-management team prescribed Celebrex. The following radiology reports will show that I have been diagnosed with several diseases attributable to the nine prostaglandin receptors. This is more than a coincidence.

I had a privileged childhood as the daughter of a new-and-used-car dealer. My father owned Fiesta Lincoln Mercury in Queens Village, New York. Does

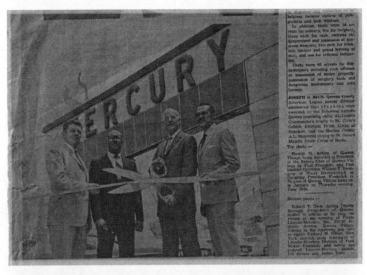

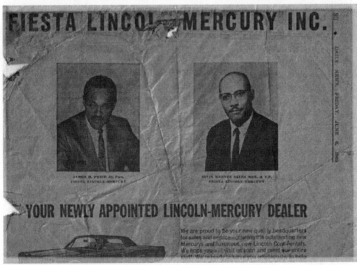

the Ford Fiesta sound familiar? The name came from my father's dealership. He was the first "Negro"/African American to own a Lincoln Mercury dealership.

My father, the handsome one on the left, started his career as a successful used-car dealer in Harlem, New York, under the name Fiesta Motors Inc. He was then offered the Lincoln Mercury franchise in Queens Village, New York, and carried the Fiesta name on from his used-car business to the Lincoln dealership. The rest is history.

As you can imagine as the daughter of the first "Negro" to own a Lincoln Mercury dealership, life was wonderful. I attended private school, and took piano and ballet lessons. I had private and timely medical care and dental treatment,

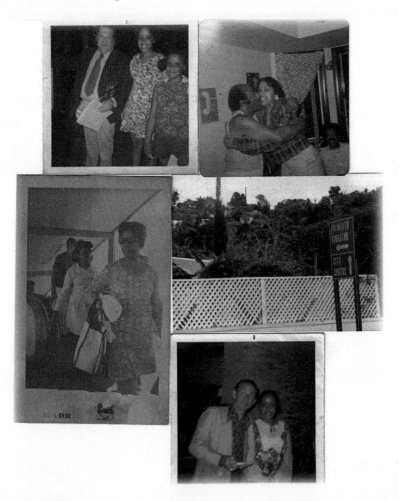

and was not exposed to environmental pollutants as I was raised in a middle-class suburban neighborhood. As a child I traveled to Europe and to the Virgin Islands, and I ate the native food. However, one can only speculate as to the source of any contamination that would have led up to the degree of illness that I am now experiencing. I rode camels in North Africa, ate pheasant in Spain, the sweetest pineapples in Puerto Rico, and seaweed-covered, sun-baked clams on the beaches of Sag Harbor, New York. I never exhibited any symptoms of illness until I became an adult. As I look back on my life, I had a normal, healthy, privileged childhood; and there was nothing that would have indicated anything was wrong.

If you look at the previous page clockwise, you'll see comedian Jackie Carter, who was performing at the hotel where I was staying in San Juan Puerto, Rico. I'm the tall one in the blue-and-white dress, and that's my baby sister, Elizabeth, next to me. Next, with my dad laughing in the background and sporting a fro while we were relaxing in Sag Harbor, New York, Roscoe Lee Brown was stealing my heart. To the bottom left, I was disembarking in Madrid, Spain. That's my cousin Cory immediately behind me. The picture next to it was taken in Jamaica, West Indies. The final picture on the bottom right is that of comedian Jackie Vernon, who was also performing at the hotel while we were on vacation in San Juan, Puerto Rico.

I did not follow any biblical principles of eating until I became a young adult. MRIs, CT scans, radiology reports, blood tests, and pathology reports don't lie. I can now only live each day, believing God that I am healed. I have learned to accept the things I cannot change and educate those that I can.

CHAPTER THREE

Sarcoid Uveitis/Iridocyclitis

It was September 1993, and the party was going full swing. Everything was going as my husband and I had planned. Our youngest son, Eric, was a year old, and the birthday boy was enjoying all the attention. I excused myself once again to check the condition of my right eye, which seemed to worsen by the hour along with my migraine headache. My eye was beet red, and any attempts to examine my eye with the sudden increase of light resulted in searing pain and tearing. I thought at that moment that perhaps I had acquired a severe infection, which had come on suddenly, perhaps conjunctivitis. At about ten that evening, I arrived at the emergency room in New York. I was not prepared for what I was about to hear.

The doctors examined me and immediately determined that what I had was not conjunctivitis. In fact, the first doctor advised me that he did not know what was wrong with my eye, but it was definitely not conjunctivitis. A specialist was called in. I waited for what seemed like an eternity. By the time the specialist arrived, my eye was almost completely shut, bright red, and felt as though someone had thrown a bag of sand in it. He examined me and began to ask me about my family history. Breathing problems? What was sarcoidosis, and why in the world was he asking me about it? Did he have the charts mixed up? I could not figure out why he was checking my breathing. What did my lungs have to do with my eyes? Every time he pointed the light in my eye, it felt as though I was being stabbed with a spear. I begged him to turn down the lights. My head felt as though it would explode. With each passing hour the pain increased. He rechecked my eye, and the direct light entering that eye caused me to let out a moan. That is when he ordered me to be transferred to their sister hospital, by ambulance. It was approximately 6:00 a.m. when I arrived. He ordered that the lights remain dim in my room. My eye pressure was checked, and several tests were performed before he made his final diagnosis. He advised me that the tests revealed my lungs were clear and my brain was fine; however, there were cells that could be seen in the anterior chamber behind the eye accompanied with flare, together with granulomatous iritis. The final diagnosis was unilateral anterior granulomatous uveitis or sarcoid uveitis. It is in the family of sarcoidosis. Topical steroids were applied, and a patch was mercifully placed over my eye to prevent light from entering. I remained legally **"blind"** for about one month. The ocular uveitis cleared up and did not return until December 10, 1994. I was in Atlanta, Georgia, for Christmas when the first symptoms recurred. The doctors at Southern Regional Medical Center concluded that since there was no conjunctival injection whatsoever, the discharge diagnosis would stand as subconjuctival hemorrhages; and they advised me to follow up with an ophthalmologist the next day as an outpatient. Needless to say, my condition worsened by the hour. My husband packed us up and drove back to New York. He had me in the emergency room by that evening. The medical records reflect that we arrived at the hospital on December 12, 1994, at 7:40 p.m. I asked for the attending physician, who initially diagnosed my condition; and, by the grace of God, he was available. To complicate matters, I was six months pregnant with my daughter. Trace cells were noted in the anterior chamber, which may account for the shorter period of temporary blindness, which was only three week's this time. Patients diagnosed with this mild form of sarcoid uveitis have decreased or hazy vision, pain in the eye, photophobia, cells and flare in the anterior chamber with granulomatous iritis.

I did have one more incident on March 1, 1995, in the right eye. A low-grade fever, swelling, redness, and mild injection of the conjunctiva of the right eye and photophobia were noted. However, it was treated early, and the condition eradicated itself quickly.

Sarcoidosis is a chronic disease that may attack almost any part of the body. It is an inflammatory disease, and tiny lumps called granulomas will grow and clump together in the infected organ. Since it is a disease involving inflammation, there is prostaglandin involvement. The most common tissue and organ involvement are the lungs, lymph nodes, eyes, skin, and liver. This systemic disease is characterized by the presence of granulated nodules in the inflamed tissue. The disease has no known cause. Patients diagnosed with sarcoidosis usually have a 20 percent incidence of ocular involvement. It usually affects the lungs and causes musculoskeletal anomalies, salivary gland infiltration, arthritis, sarcoid nodules of the skin, tuberculosis-like inflammation, with cough and fatigue. The interesting thing about sarcoidosis is that it may progress and worsen, or it may disappear completely. The clinical features of sarcoidosis are also known to mimic rheumatologic diseases, which make the onset of the next series of events in my life very interesting.

OPHTHALMOLOGY
CLINIC RECORD

F. 34 yo old.

Price Stacey
Brown 74 - 65 - 97

HOLY FAMILY HOME   ST. JOHN'S QUEENS
MARY IMMACULATE   ST. JOSEPH'S
MSGR. FITZPATRICK   ST. MARY'S HOSPITAL OF BROOKLYN

34 yo BOT

Present Complaint: Evaluated @ SA. Svc 10/1/93   Date: 10/8/93
@ Eye pain + Extreme photophobia

Past Ocular History: ATC c̄ similar complaints
@ 7 Days PF 1% OD @ cyclog.

Past Medical History: Migrane HA.
w/ MRI CT 9/93.

Allergy: NKDA.

Medications: 1. Ophthalmic – PF 1% 4/o.

2. Other —

Vdsc 20/40 +1 ph 20/20 **Vdcc** ph Wd Fd Md
20/15 –

Vnsc ph **Vncc** Wn Mn

motility: full

pupils: 3/3mm 3/3T ⊕ APD.

confrontation fields: Grossly n OS, Restricted

lids and lashes: wnl OU

conjunctiva: 2+ Inj/chem OD

cornea: wnl OU

anterior chamber: 4+ cells/flare OD

iris: wnl OU

tension: OD: Sft OS: Soft   time: 1215°

DILATED EXAM

lens:

vitreous: wnl per dx – 10/1/93

fundus:

LABORATORY STUDIES:

ASSESSMENT/PLAN: ① Iritocyclitis
↑ Pred Forte Q 1° ⊕ ×
cyclog T ↑ OD Q FE

Return date: ATC 5 Day   meds renewed c̄ MID.   **Referral to:** OD c̄ Dr ____ c̄ Dr ____ M.D! F/u

Side 1

```
RICARDO              , M.D.          | Excuse slip from:
   UPPER RIVERDALE ROAD              | RICARDO            M.D.
SUITE #100                           |    UPPER RIVERDALE ROAD
RIVERDALE         GA 30274           | RIVERDALE         GA 30274
                                     | Phone:
Telephone  770                       | Patient: STACEY      BROWN
                                     | Date:     04/27/00
                                     | Time:     10:58 AM
```

```
   Bill to AI0015866                              For Patient

     STACEY     P BROWN


                            GA 30297
```

| Date of | Product/ | | | | Insurance | Patient |
Service	Service	Description		Qty	Amount	Amount

```
       ***** BILL # 157540  BILL DATE 02/07/00
02/07/00 92014    COMPREHENSIVE ESTABLISHED EXAM           1
   DIAGNOSIS=364.02 RECURRENT IRIDOCYCLITIS
   DIAGNOSIS=135    SARCOIDOSIS
03/03/00 PER PRUDENTIAL NEED INFORMATION REGARDING ANOTHER
03/03/00 COVERAGE. RELEASED TO PATIENT W/COPY OF INS EOB
03/17/00 PER NDC CLAIM FORWARDED TO PRUDENTIAL
04/11/00        Adjustment HMO ADJUSTMENT
04/11/00        Payment--PRUDENTIAL HEALTHCAR
                                               BAL DUE

                                        Total Due
```

```
Attended by              Fed ID #     BC/BS #   State License #
RICARDO        , M.D.
```

```
. . . . . . . . . . . . . . . . . . . . . .
| PLEASE MAKE CHECKS PAYABLE TO      |
| CENTER.             JA 30358.*     |
| ALL CREDIT CARDS ACCEPTED. ANY QUESTION. |
| PLEASE CALL OUR BILLING DEPARTMENT AT 770 - |
. . . . . . . . . . . . . . . . . . . . . .
```

```
Your next appointment is on
            MON  May 08, 2000      AT 08:45AM
               UPPER RIVERDALE RD #100
               RIVERDALE         GA 30274
```

The doctor's name and address were deleted to protect his privacy.

Iridocyclitis is a disease whereby the uvea of the eye suffers inflammation. The symptoms include photophobia, redness, watering of the eyes, and blurred vision. Chronic iridocyclitis is associated with systemic disorders: ankylosing spondylitis, Behcet's syndrome, inflammatory bowel disease, sarcoidosis, syphilis, juvenile rheumatoid arthritis, Reiter's syndrome, tuberculosis, and Lyme disease. Iridocyclitis is classified as an autoimmune disease. The cause of my disease was diagnosed as sarcoidosis/sarcoid uveitis. If this disease is left untreated, it has been statistically the third leading cause of preventable blindness in the world. **Most ophthalmologists are not trained in the diagnosis and treatment of this rare disease (Uveitis.org)**. In the illustration below, the uvea is located between the

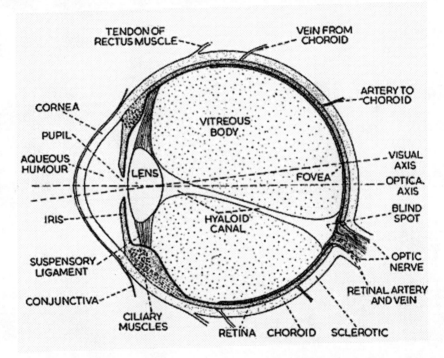

cornea and the retina. When the uvea becomes inflamed, it develops lymphocytic infiltrates resulting in uveitis.

The following is an illustration of what the eye chamber looks like after it becomes inflamed and the granulomas are visible on film. It is a fact that some individuals have a genetic predisposition to uveitis related to an autoimmune disease process. Multiple sclerosis, idiopathic arthritis, and sarcoidosis have all been linked to recurrent uveitis. However, what is the likelihood of someone having **all** these aforementioned diseases? I do!

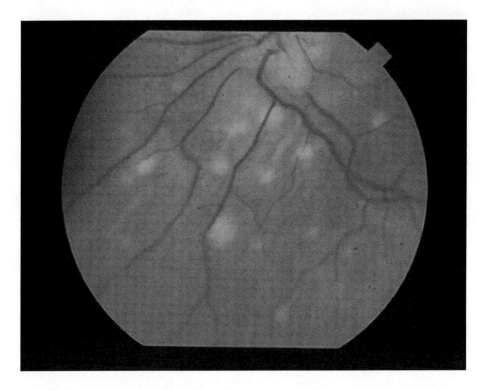

Ocular Uveitis/Iridocyclitis (The white spots in the film are the granulomas.)

CHAPTER FOUR

Right Hand/First Digit

Prior to the diagnosis in 1993 of sarcoid uveitis, my right hand had always given me trouble, and I never knew why. In law school, it would fall asleep while I was writing. I would wake up in the morning, and my right hand would be swollen. While playing golf, my arms would go numb, but I was determined to keep up with the boys and show off my good game, not to mention my pink outfit, matching golf bag, shoes, and cover. Especially with all the attention and help I was getting with my swing, it was easier to ignore the mild discomfort. The condition would resolve itself quickly and was usually explained away by overexertion. It was not until the connection was made to the sarcoidosis that the pieces to the medical puzzle began to fit. I was a heavy smoker, approximately one pack a day. After the death of my father in 1988, my smoking took on a feverish pitch and escalated to approximately two packs a day and didn't stop until January 1998. My mother in law had a nickname for me—Chimney—because I smoked like one and must have smelled like one too. She didn't tell me about it until after I stopped smoking, but she prayed for me. We still laugh about it today. Evidently, prayer works!

In or around 1991 or 1992, my right hand was continuously swollen and numb. At times, the whole right arm would lose circulation, but the loss of circulation and pain was primarily confined to the right hand. In 1992, something interesting happened. The first digit on my right hand took on a life all its own. It turned completely gray, black, and blue in color, and began to twist and swell; and the nail bed began to deform. It literally began to form ridges and turned black in color. The color change was not sudden. It seemed to increase with the pain and swelling. The knuckle, to this day, is anthropoid in appearance. The anthropoid appearance is attributed to osteoarthritis. When the nail bed turned completely black, I sought help. A biopsy revealed noncaseating granulomas consistent with sarcoidosis. I will never forget the biopsy. It was localized anesthesia, and a scalpel was placed underneath the nail bed, removing a significant portion of the nail and flesh. I bled profusely and still felt pain in spite of the doctor's efforts to neutralize the pain.

The first line of therapy is prednisone or other systemic treatments like colchicines. I have seen what steroids do to people, and I know what they have done to me. They are extremely addictive and cause excessive weight gain. A doctor prescribed high doses of medication, which resulted in an allergic reaction resulting in a rash, swelling, and only temporarily relieved the pain and inflammation. The right digit remained twisted, blue, gray, black, and swollen. I continued to seek other medical opinions and assistance, and I was afraid to try other drugs; but looking at the condition of my finger I had little choice. I tried various combinations of drugs, and that's when I discovered I am allergic to NSAIDS and Robaxin. I became desperate and was even willing to try radical methods to return my right index finger to normal. I sought the opinion of an

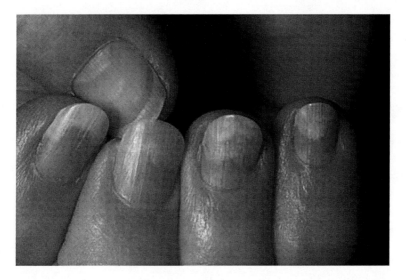

This is what a hand looks like after it has been infected with sarcoidosis lesions.

oncologist and a radiologist for consideration of palliative radiotherapy to the right hand. My hand could have been used in a sci-fi feature; it was so horribly disfigured. The pain in my hand was unbearable, and I was willing to try radiation therapy to the first digit of my right hand to a dose of 1000 cGy at 200 cGy per fraction using mega voltage x-rays. Medical literature reports excellent results for radiation therapy for neurosarcoidosis at a dose of 3000 cGy at 300 Gy per fraction, but the literature is scant for bony involvement of sarcoid. Although there is a 1 in 10,000 chance of developing sarcoma, bone cancer, the risk would have been well taken in light of the benefit. After thinking it over, I decided not to undergo the radiation therapy for my finger, but the pain and swelling continued; and I was back where I started.

PATIENT: BROWN, STACEY   . DATE: 9/15/95

REFERRING PHYSICIAN: Paul _____ |M.D.

CONSULTING PHYSICIAN: John _____ |, M.D.

PROFILE:

This is a 36 year old woman with a history of sarcoidosis referred
for consideration of palliative radiotherapy to the right hand.

CONCLUSIONS:

1. Diagnosed as having sarcoidosis in 1993.
2. History of anterior uveitis secondary to sarcoidosis, treated
    with topical steroids.
3. History of chronic right first digit pain secondary to
    sarcoidosis, biopsied at the
    New York.
4. Absolute refusal of prednisone or colchicine.

RECOMMENDATION:

To deliver radiation therapy to the right first digit to a dose of
1000 cGy at 200 cGy per fraction using megavoltage x-rays.

ASSESSMENT:

This is a 36 year old black woman who reportedly in 1993, was
diagnosed as having sarcoidosis. At that time, she was noted to
have mediastinal adenopathy and right hilar adenopathy on chest x-
ray. Reportedly she refused diagnostic procedures to the chest.
In September of 1993, she developed bilateral anterior uveitis and
temporary loss of vision. She was treated in New York for
sarcoidosis involving the uvea with topical steroids. Her vision
improved. Intermittently since that time she has had progressive
right hand pain, especially in the right first digit. She had a
biopsy of the right first digit in 1994 and reportedly this
revealed noncaseating granulomas consistent with sarcoidosis. We
are obtaining these records from Long Island, NY. She has
adamantly refused first line therapy of Prednisone or other
systemic treatments like Colchicine. She has been taking Darvocet
for her intermittent right hand pain. She recently noted bilateral
lower extremity pain as well. She denies any headache, recent
visual changes or balance problems. She denies any persistent
cough, fever, or chest pain. She denies any abdominal pain or
changes in bladder or rectal function. Recent chest x-ray
performed on 6/20/95 reveals normal mediastinal and hilar
structures and no evidence of interstitial disease.

(cont.)

On physical exam, in general, she is a well appearing black woman
in no acute distress. HEENT: normocephalic, atraumatic.
Extraocular muscles are intact. Pupils are equal, round, and
reactive to light. Neck showed some shotty adenopathy in the left
lower neck. Axillary areas revealed a 1 cm left axillary lymph
node. Right axilla was negative. Lungs showed some minor
inspiratory wheezing. Cardiovascular exam showed a regular rate
and rhythm. Abdomen was flat with no palpable masses. The liver
was palpated 3 cm below the right costophrenic angle. The spleen
was normal in size. Groins were negative. Extremities showed some
edema of the right first digit, especially around the distal
interphalangeal joint and proximal interphalangeal joint. Her
finger was markedly tender to palpation. She had good range of
motion. Her bilateral lower extremities were tender to palpation,
especially in the anterior tibia region. No other clubbing,
cyanosis or edema was noted. Neurologically, motor, sensory and
cerebellar exam were grossly intact.

DISCUSSION:

This is a 36 year old woman with a history of sarcoidosis producing
transient blindness secondary to anterior uveitis as well as
apparent bony involvement of the right first digit producing
significant pain. Of course the first line therapy is Prednisone
and then possibly Colchicine. She adamantly refuses any systemic
therapy for this disease. She presents today for consideration of
radiation to the right first digit. Of course, the literature is
very scant as far as radiation for sarcoidosis. Bejar, et al, and
Grizaanti, et al, have reported on treating the whole brain for
neurosarcoidosis refractory to prednisone. Fogel has reported on
treating the larynx for also refractory sarcoidosis. They report
good results with 3000 cGy at 300 cGy per fraction. We are
searching the medical literature for radiation therapy for bony
involvement of sarcoid. I have agreed to treat Mrs. Brown but she
has been thoroughly informed as to the limited data for radiation
therapy for this disease. The side effects including minor skin
changes, injury to the PIP and DIP joints as well as the risk of 1
in 10,000 of developing any secondary malignancy including sarcoma
was discussed with Mrs. Brown. She has given informed consent. We
will keep you informed.

John   M.D.
Radiation Oncologist

JHG:rw
cc: Paul   M.D.

CHAPTER FIVE

Osteoarthritis

Osteoarthritis or degenerative arthritis is a disease of the joints, and is caused by the breakdown and eventual loss of cartilage of one or more joints. As the body continues to age, the water content of the cartilage decreases, and the protein makeup of the cartilage degenerates. Repetitive use of the joints irritates and inflames the cartilage, causing joint pain and swelling. Over time the cartilage will begin to degenerate by flaking and forming tiny crevasses. When the degeneration is severe, there is total loss of cartilage between the bones of the joints, leading to friction, pain, and limitation of joint mobility. Repeated friction and inflammation of the cartilage can lead to the growth of new bone outgrowth called spurs. Obesity, trauma, gout, diabetes, and hormone disorders are factors that have been attributed to this condition. This condition is what is known as secondary osteoarthritis. The difference between osteoarthritis and rheumatoid arthritis is that osteoarthritis is a disease that does not affect other organs of the body. A systemic illness is a disease that will affect other organs of the body, and osteoarthritis is a disease that is limited to the joints found in the hands, spine, feet, hips, and knees (large weight-bearing joints). Unless there is a diagnosis of secondary osteoarthritis, then there is no known cause and, as in my case, the diagnosis is primary osteoarthritis. Most medical professionals attribute this condition to aging and repetitive use of the joints in the absence of any evidence of trauma. For example, early onset is attributed in athletes such as weight lifters and soccer players. The constant impact to the knees and joint tissue can cause early onset of osteoarthritis.

There are over one hundred different types of arthritis conditions, and osteoarthritis is the most common. Statistically, males are affected before they reach age forty-five and women after they reach fifty-five. Loss of cartilage cushion causes friction between the bones and naturally causes pain and limitation of mobility. Eventually, cartilage degeneration can lead to deformity. The combination of degeneration and weight gain on the knee will result in the knee bowing out. As a result, the knee will have to be replaced. This is a result of the complications associated with secondary osteoarthritis and weight gain. Minus the weight gain, complete loss of the cartilage cushion will result in extreme pain and will cause joint dysfunction and eventual limping. Osteoarthritis of the spine results in bone spurs forming along the spine that irritates the spinal nerves, causing severe pain, numbness, and tingling. The neck and low back are affected more than any other part of the spine.

Osteoarthritis also affects the formation of the hard bony enlargement of the small joints of the fingers. The joints begin to deform as a result of the bone spurs from the Osteoarthritis in the joint.

Osteoarthritis is diagnosed as a matter of exclusion. There is no blood test for this disease, so the doctor will determine the findings based on a positive bone spurring and joint space narrowing in the x-rays, in addition to a negative finding for other systemic diseases.

My blood tests were negative for rheumatoid arthritis, but my x-rays were positive for osteoarthritis in the hands and spine. It is common among African Americans to have rheumatoid arthritis, which is a systemic, crippling, and deadly form of arthritis.

The knuckle on my right digit is anthropoid in appearance due to inflammation and swelling in the joint caused by disease. I can remember having this condition since my days in college. The finger next to it just doesn't seem to fit quite comfortably into the socket. Extreme cold and "use," such as simple housework, causes pain and swelling in the affected area. In my lifetime I do not recall any trauma to the right hand as I led a pretty sedentary life and was not involved in any injury. Even schoolwork caused my hand to swell. I love gardening, writing, golf, gourmet cooking, playing the piano, and enjoying my chosen profession, law, until disease and time claimed my ability to actively engage in these activities. Then my doctor prescribed Vioxx, the miracle drug. It had no known side effects, and I took the drug as prescribed from around December 1999 or January 2000 to June of 2000. The reason my doctor stopped prescribing it was that a tumor began to form at the base of my brain. It was sticking out of the back of my neck. He ordered a gastrointestinal exam, a colonoscopy, and began monitoring my blood pressure more than usual. I couldn't understand the reason for these procedures and began to question him. This agitated him, and he refused any explanation; so I adamantly refused to comply with the in office colonoscopy, and as such our doctor-patient relationship ended. He also did not understand that I was afraid to have the colonoscopy procedure in his office and that I would have preferred a hospital setting. I did not connect the dots until the Vioxx lawsuits hit the media. I was referred to a neurosurgeon to have the mass removed, and I ended up at Piedmont Hospital Medical Group.

When I filed a suit, he refused to cooperate with my attorneys and did not turn over my medical records. At the end of the day, my medical records suddenly

June 8, 2005

Ms. Stacey Price Brown

Re: **YOUR VIOXX, BEXTRA AND/OR CELEBREX CASE**

Dear Stacey:

      We appreciate your confidence in hiring our law firm to represent you concerning your exposure to potentially dangerous medications. It is very important that we document your use of the medication so we can determine the extent of your exposure and its impact on your physical condition.

      We would like to ask that you please obtain from your pharmacist a copy of a list of prescriptions filled and forward them to our   office to the attention of my Paralegal,   I would also request that if you have any medical records and/or bills that relate to problems with your medication use, for example, hospital visits for heart attacks, strokes, high blood pressure, stomach problems and blood clotting, that you forward those to our office as well.

      If there are any individuals that are currently applying for Social Security benefits or have been disabled by a Personal Injury claim or a Workers' Compensation claim, I would ask that you please contact my Paralegal,   to inform her of this matter.

      I appreciate your assistance and will keep you posted as further legal development concerning your case arise.

Respectfully yours,

Attorney at Law

RRP/smh

ATTORNEYS

June 8, 2005

Ms. Stacey Price Brown

Re: **YOUR VIOXX, BEXTRA AND/OR CELEBREX CASE**

Dear Stacey:

We appreciate your confidence in hiring our law firm to represent you concerning your exposure to potentially dangerous medications. It is very important that we document your use of the medication so we can determine the extent of your exposure and its impact on your physical condition.

We would like to ask that you please obtain from your pharmacist a copy of a list of prescriptions filled and forward them to our   office to the attention of my Paralegal,   I would also request that if you have any medical records and/or bills that relate to problems with your medication use, for example, hospital visits for heart attacks, strokes, high blood pressure, stomach problems and blood clotting, that you forward those to our office as well.

If there are any individuals that are currently applying for Social Security benefits or have been disabled by a Personal Injury claim or a Workers' Compensation claim. I would ask that you please contact my Paralegal,   to inform her of this matter.

I appreciate your assistance and will keep you posted as further legal development concerning your case arise.

Respectfully yours,

Attorney at Law

RRP/smh

LAW OFFICES OF   **P.C.**

ATTORNEYS AT LAW

August 17, 2006

WITHDRAWAL OF REPRESENTATION

Dear Stacey - Brown :

       Please allow this letter to serve as this Law Firm's notice of withdrawal of representing you on your individual Vioxx, Bextra and /or Celebrex case. Recent decisions in court cases in New Jersey and California concerning the medication Vioxx indicate that only certain cases involving heart attack and stroke will prevail against the Merck Corporation which makes Vioxx. These decisions have been rendered since our Law Firm began representation of you on potential claim. We believe that these same restrictions may apply to Celebrex and Bextra users. This has required this Law Firm to restrict our representation of clients to just these small categories.

       Additionally, this Law Firm has not been selected by the Federal Courts to represent the Class Action cases that are being filed or will be filed in the near future. Your interest may be protected by one of these Law Firms. I am strongly going to recommend that you consult another Law Firm concerning your rights to file an individual lawsuit and to opt out of the the class action lawsuit.

       There is a statute of limitations as to the filing of individual claim against the Merck Corporation for Vioxx use. The last date that lawsuit may be filed with the Federal Court is in September 29th, 2006 The statute of limitations for the filing of individual claims against Pfizer Corporation which makes Bextra and Celebrex is potentially April 5th 2007. I will again strongly recommend if you wish to file an individual claim, that you consult another Law Firm to determine your rights.

       I wanted to conclude by saying that this Notice of Withdrawal from filing an individual claim does not affect your right to participate in the Class Action Lawsuits that will or have been filed. Additionally, this notice does not affect any other claim which this Law Firm may be representing you on. We will continue to represent your interests on those cases. Please feel free to contact our offices concerning this matter.

                             Respectfully,

                             Attorney at Law

disappeared. My attorneys had to get proof that I took the drug for the prescribed period of time from my insurance company, which was all that was required to file a suit and proof that I was "injured permanently" under the terms of the law. These circumstances, in and of itself, were suspect. I personally went to his office and asked for my medical records, and was refused. I was told he was with patients and that I had to pay for the records and that they had to be copied. At first he wanted fifty dollars for the file, and, of course, my attorney agreed to this. Then his office could not produce the records because his office claimed the file was in storage and that we had to wait. Then his office claimed he was on vacation. After waiting another three weeks and not returning any of my calls, personal visits, or my attorneys' calls, they claimed they had the medical file; but we had

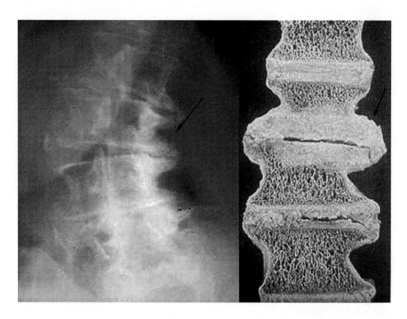

to wait for the file to be copied. After three months of this, we got the message that he was not going to turn over my records or that, in the alternative, the file had been destroyed. We contacted my insurance carrier responsible for handling the claim. After contacting their legal department and explaining the doctor's behavior, their microfiche records were turned over to my attorneys' office so that we could finally proceed with filing the lawsuit. Even after all this, the attorney decided to withdraw representation with only a few days left in the statutory period to file, and the excuse was that I did not have a heart attack or a stroke and that my "injury" was unlike the class of the other victims'. However, I ask you to view the results of the drug trials enumerated in chapter 32. Based on the foregoing information, I ask that you be the judge and the jury. As a result of taking Vioxx and Celebrex, it set off a series of events that resulted in my now having several rare diseases. It literally caused a genetic breakdown.

The following are actual x-rays of the spine illustrating the effects of osteoarthritis. Note the darkened areas in the x-rays. These show areas of desiccation. The next series of x-rays show the actual progression: loss of disc height, cord compression, disc spurring, loss of signal, etc. If I didn't know better, I would think I was looking at my own x-rays! My favorite analogy of my spine is driving a car and trying to stop without brake pads.

This is essentially what my right hand looks like as a result of osteoarthritis. The raised anthropoid knuckles and the index and middle fingers appear to be disfigured from the affects of osteoarthritis.

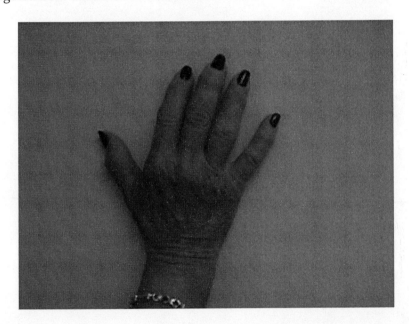

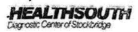
HEALTHSOUTH
Diagnostic Center of Stockbridge

STACY BROWN #30232
APRIL 22, 2002
PAGE 2

IMPRESSION: Degenerative disc disease with mild spondylosis from C3 to C6 without significant neural compressive effect, but with cord impingement or indentation at each level of relatively minor degree.

C6-7: Left paracentral superiorly and inferiorly extruded herniation with left-sided cord flattening and left C7 nerve root irritation.

DANIEL G. SCHWARTZBERG, M.D.

DGS/vlo
Transcribed: 4/23/02

7384 Hannover Parkway S. Suite 100 • Stockbridge, CA 30281 • 678 289-0707 • fax 678 289-0708

CHAPTER SIX

Brain Tumor
(The following is a clear example of
tumorigenisis.)

When one thinks of the brain, we immediately think of it as a single bulbous organ encased in the skull and responsible for our thought processes. However, the brain is responsible for our life processes. It receives a steady stream of information and signals to the other body organs. Our emotions begin in the brain so the brain controls love, hate, fear, and anger. If we are hungry or thirsty, our brain tells us to eat or drink. The brain is very complex and can also store memories from past experiences and will plan future events. The brain can learn and adapt, and it can remember. The brain enables man to speak and to solve problems. The brain is not a single organ but is made up of many parts with specific functions.

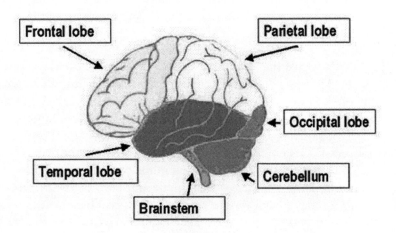

Many tiny blood vessels are needed to feed the brain. Remember the prostaglandin receptor acting on the spinal cord causing pain and affecting the central nervous system? Examples of diseases of the brain are tumors and multiple sclerosis. The brain communicates within itself, if you will, by a system set up with billions of tiny neurons, each consisting of cell bodies connected to other cell bodies. Each neuron has fine branching fibers at one end called dendrites. A single dendrite fiber is called an axon. Many bundles of axons are called white matter. Impulses are received over the axon, and as such there is cell to cell communication. Neurons are the main cells that carry out the brain's functions. The nerve cell bodies and the surrounding mesh of fibers are called gray matter. Gray matter is made up of the core of the spinal cord and its upward extension into the base of the brain, which is called the brain stem.

The three main divisions in the brain are the forebrain, the midbrain, and the hindbrain. So let me break it down for you. The front of the skull contains the cerebrum, which is the largest part of the brain. It has two halves, which are called left and right hemispheres. The hemispheres communicate with each other by a bundle of nerves called corpus callosum. The folds that you see in the brain are actually a thin carpet of nerve cells called the cerebral cortex or gray matter, which covers the cerebrum. The folding allows the brain to fit within the limited space in the skull. Beneath the cortex is white matter. They are nerve fibers connecting the cortex to the brain stem. The groups of nerve cells within the white matter are called basil ganglia. It is the largest and the most important part of the brain because it accounts for our intelligence. It can be divided into three parts and is responsible for our emotions, regulating body function such as hunger and thirst, and it acts in concert with the midbrain to control the reticular system. The midbrain is responsible for the reticular system, and this is what keeps us awake and alert.

Each hemisphere of the cerebrum is divided into five lobes, and they are named for the bones of the skull: frontal, temporal, parietal, and occipital. The limbic lobe is in the middle of the cerebrum where the hemispheres face each other. One of the most important parts of the brain is the sensorimotor area. It is located on each side of the central fissure and sends nerve impulses to the muscle used for skilled movement such as playing the piano, throwing a ball, playing golf, etc. Each hemisphere controls different parts of the body. The upper part of the sensorimotor controls a leg, the middle part controls an arm, and the lower part controls the muscles of the tongue and face. It involves touch and sends sensory messages from various parts of the body. These messages include pressure, sensation, and things that we take for granted like movement. Incoming and outgoing pathways to the sensory area cross in the brain stem.

Did you ever wonder how we hear? The ear sends messages to the temporal lobe just below the central fissure. The temporal lobe is contained in the cerebral cortex, and it is responsible for speech, thought, and memories. Speech is also located in parts of the frontal and parietal lobes. The occipital lobe receives impulses from the eyes and allows us to see, form pictures, and directs the movement of our eyes.

The diencephalon of the forebrain has three main parts, which control the activities of a person's body. They are the hypothalamus (which controls hunger, thirst, temperature) and the pituitary gland. It also controls fear and anger and the reticular system, which is responsible for keeping the brain awake and alert. The subthalamus, as its name would indicate, is responsible for coordinating movements. It contains many fibers that carry impulses from the basil ganglia to the thalamus and from the thalamus to the hypothalamus. The thalamus relays sensory impulses from the cerebellum to the cerebral cortex.

The midbrain can be found between the diencephalon and the medulla oblongata. Its function is to control movements of the eyes and other parts of the body, and it plays an important part in the reticular system. Beneath the midbrain is a bulblike formation called pons. Their function is to act as a relay sending sensory impulses between the cerebrum and cerebellum.

The term medulla oblongata refers to the oblong extension of the spinal cord into the back of the head. It begins at the base of the skull, continues upward, and forms the lower part of the brain stem. If you splice a telephone cord that is pretty much the same way your nerve fibers are bundled in the medulla. The medulla contains nerve centers that control swallowing, breathing, muscle tone, heartbeat, blood flow, posture, movement of the stomach and intestines. It has centers connected with the organs of balance in the ears. The reticular system is a network of nerves that lies between the nerve center of the medulla and extends upward into higher levels of the brain stem and extend down the spinal cord. Its function is to keep the brain alert and to assist in coordinating and regulating brain function.

The base of the brain is called the cerebellum. It regulates posture, movement, and balance, and controls the position and movement of the body according to what is seen and heard. One must immediately think of a blind person. As such, the position and movement will be controlled by what is heard because it works automatically as do many areas of the brain.

If the brain is damaged, these functions may be impaired. The most common type of damage is a clot or tumor. A brain tumor may damage the brain. Once the tumor is removed, any part of the brain that is removed cannot be replaced. Further, any damage to brain cells is also permanent because brain cells do not grow back. Once cells are damaged, others take over the work of the lost or damaged cells; but it is never the same. Once the cerebellum is damaged, a person will have difficulty moving their arms and legs. There are many diseases that affect the brain. Multiple sclerosis is an autoimmune disease and is a disease of the central nervous system, which scars the brain and may eventually affect the whole body and its ability to function properly. We are also familiar with aneurysm, cerebral hemorrhage, and cerebral palsy, just to name a few. A virus or high fever can affect the brain or a common disease such as the mumps or measles, vitamin deficiency, or diabetes. The brain is so complex it is difficult to determine the extent of injury once the brain has been damaged from disease or injury. The brain continually gives off small waves of electricity. Wires can be attached to the scalp, and electrically driven pens record the waves on continuously moving strips of paper. This record is called an electroencephalogram, or an EEG.

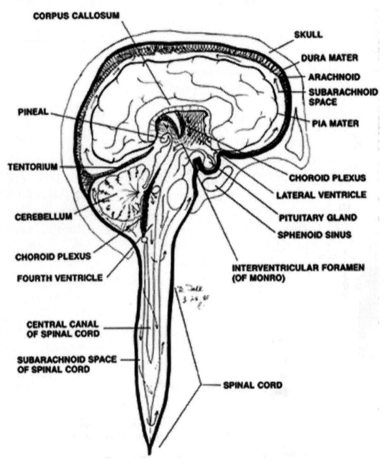

The brain still holds many mysteries for scientists, and the biggest one is behavior. Behavior is defined as how one makes judgments and decisions or plans for future actions. Since the beginning of time, we have tried to put a name on the way we behave. Good versus evil. Man has structured the way we act in varied and succinct doctrines called religion. It is the way we justify the way we act. Religion is the basis of our moral fiber and God-given free will up to a point. Society restricted that free will by imposing laws. Man tried to figure out thought and action by inventing psychiatrists; but like any form of medicine it is a practice, and it has its benefits, and it is also flawed.

After taking Vioxx for approximately six months, a tumor began to grow between my medulla oblongata and the cervical spine, affecting the bundle of nerves and the right side of my body. It was quite an unusual tumor because it was sticking out of the back of my head. The circulation in my right arm and leg was affected. It was hard to the touch. As a matter of fact, it actually bounced if you hit it just right. It was something that was quite unusual, a tumor growing out of the back of the neck like a dinosaur horn; so naturally, fear was my reaction. Now I had this unfamiliar, painful, hard thing growing out of the base of my brain that moved to the touch—and it hurt. With all my other medical problems, this one rose to the top of the "to do" list. I had to do something about this fast. I consulted with a neurosurgeon because the pain was now at an unbearable level. After consultation and examination, a neurosurgeon at Piedmont Hospital scheduled surgery for November 9, 2000.

Before going into surgery I had to prepare myself. I got my house in order, and my mother arrived from Florida to help me with my children; but I needed to be prepared mentally because I was a basket case. James 4:16 tells us, "Is any sick among you? Let him call for the elders of the church; and let them pray over him, anointing him with oil in the name of the Lord." So I went to church. My pastor and the elders of the church anointed me, and I prayed till the sun came up and went down again. I marched into surgery like a true soldier of the Lord. When it was time for the operating room nurse to mark the back of my neck for the sight of the tumor, she acted as if she saw a ghost. She stammered and went for the surgeon. I believe that huge lump sticking out of the back of my head might have startled her. I looked like a human version of a dinosaur of sorts. **God showed up and showed out**; a miracle took place that day. The tumor was sitting up and sticking out, which made it easier for it to be removed. I was out of surgery in less than the estimated time.

The radiology report stated that a chrondroma or a benign cartilaginous growth as well as herniated intervertebral disc material was removed from the interspinous region of the cervical spine. The report further indicated that it was a hard single mass of white solid tissue. The shape was irregular but was delivered to the pathologist in two pieces, and the sizes were indicated as follows: 1.5 x 1.0 x 0.5 cm and 1.4 x 0.7 x 0.5 cm. When you think about the size and shape of the average neck of an average woman and given all the things that are contained therein, that was a pretty sizeable tumor; and I was glad to be rid of it. My circulation almost immediately returned to normal. However, there remains significant disc herniation at C6-C7 with spinal cord compression due to degenerative disc disease.

Just to refresh our memories, the prostaglandin receptor acting on spinal neurons causes pain. Neurons are **cells** that can be found in the **brain, spinal** cord, nerves, and ganglia of the peripheral nervous system. They transmit electrical signals and are a major class of cells found in the nervous system. Another prostaglandin affects **calcium movement** in the body. The tumor was described as a chondroma, and clinical correlation was recommended; however, the neurologist, pain management specialist, psychiatrist never followed up! The exact medical terminology is chondroblastoma or Codman's tumor. It is an extremely **rare benign bone tumor** in that it most often affects the ends of the long bones of the arms and legs at the hip, shoulder, and knee. So then the

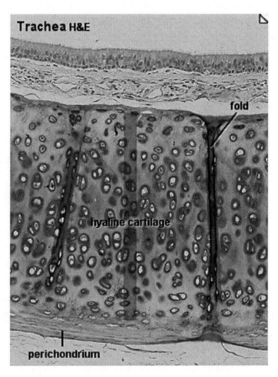

This is what hyaline cartilage looks like.

question that immediately comes to mind is, What was it doing at the base of the brain, at the medulla oblongata, as a posterior cervical mass?

The interesting thing about the pathology report is that it contained benign hyaline cartilage. Although it is semitransparent, it contains **living cells and chondrocytes.** Hyaline cartilage is responsible for the longitudinal growth of bone in the neck regions of the long bones. The C-shaped hyaline cartilage rings also assists in keeping the trachea and bronchi tubes open.

It took approximately six weeks for me to heal from the surgery. I believe I recovered quickly because I was anxious to resume a "normal" routine in light of the postsurgical conditions. I did enjoy a brief vacation from caring for my children. Thank God for mothers. I was not able to raise my arms above my chest or scratch my nose. You know the old saying, "You don't miss what you have until it's gone." Well, the full range of motion and the strength in my arms were gone, and I couldn't wash or comb my hair, and I could barely brush my teeth. No one would attempt to comb it for me, so you can imagine what my hair looked and smelled like. I wore the sorriest-looking ponytail for weeks. My husband and mother did, however, change my bandages. I was used to washing and conditioning my hair every few days and bathing daily. I was not able to get the incision wet because of the risk of infection, so my husband gave me a sponge bath. There is something to be said about a man who is that caring and loving, and there is a great degree of sensuality in a sponge bath when the right amount of time and care is taken. So I guess the recovery period wasn't so bad after all, and I do have fond memories of those sponge baths.

PIEDMONT HOSPITAL
PROMINA 1968 PEACHTREE ROAD, N.W. • ATLANTA, GA 30309

Mark H. DuPuis, M.D.
DIRECTOR OF LABORATORY

Patient Name:	**BROWN, STACEY PATRICE**	*Accession #:*	**PS-00-016068**
Patient #:	00305-90396	*Admit Date:*	11/09/2000
Med. Rec. #:	(00001)0-002124569	*Location:*	0501 - 01
Birth Date:	05/23/1959 *Age:* 41 YRS *Sex:* F	*Discharged:*	11/10/2000
Request Doctor:		*Collect Date:*	11/09/00
Admit Doctor:		*Service Date:*	11/09/00
Consult. Doctor:		*Print Date:*	11/17/00 1538

Copy To:

SURGICAL PATHOLOGY REPORT

FINAL DIAGNOSIS:

Soft tissue mass, posterior neck, excision
 - benign hyaline cartilage and fibrocartilaginous tissue, see comment

COMMENT: Benign hyaline cartilage and fibrocartilage are present associated
with skeletal muscle and fibroadipose connective tissue. The differential
diagnosis is felt to include benign cartilaginous lesions such as chondroma of
soft tissue as well as herniated intervertebral disc material. Clinical
correlation is recommended. There is no evidence of malignancy.

CLINICAL INFORMATION:
Posterior cervical mass

GROSS DESCRIPTION:
The specimen is labeled "posterior neck mass." Received in formalin are two
irregular pieces of hard, white solid tissue, 1.5 x 1.0 x 0.5 cm and 1.4 x 0.7
x 0.5 cm. ES

11/09/00   By: PTT / HLH

SLIDE INDEX:
1A - entire specimen

SLIDE BLOCK TALLY:
1 H+E section

Transcribed Final: 11/10/00 BFW/EAN
Verified by:_____ 11/10/00
                          M.D.   /BFW
          (Electronic Signature)

<<< End of Report >>>   *Page: 1*

CHAPTER SEVEN

Raynaud's Phenomenon vs. Vasculitis

It was December 1994, and I am pregnant with my third child. We decided to relocate from New York to Georgia because of the milder climate, and Georgia was where we wanted to raise our growing family. We arrived in Georgia December 1994, and no sooner than I arrived, I was welcomed with a virus that apparently had been active in the home where we had been invited to stay. Everyone got sick, and I ended up in the emergency room two weeks before Christmas—pregnant and with the flu. A week later I went blind in my left eye and had to return to New York for treatment. After all the excitement, we finally settled down in a rented town home two months before we purchased our home. We had a wonderful Christmas with new friends. We were truly blessed. I thought everything had finally calmed down until about mid-December when we were grocery shopping and I went into labor. After I was released from the hospital, I was immediately put on bed rest. Although I was put on bed rest, I still had a four—and two-year-old to take care of while my husband was at work. The swelling increased with use such as ordinary housework. Not only was there lack of circulation in my arms, but there was lack of circulation and pain in my legs as well. My pregnancy was considered high risk because of my age and medical history. It is common during pregnancy for a woman's feet to swell, but my hands were swollen too. My unborn daughter continued to try to arrive before her birthday, so I was placed on bed rest and medication to prevent her untimely arrival. My beautiful daughter was born at thirty-seven weeks on February 20, 1995. She refused to stay, and there was nothing the doctors could do because she broke my water and was delivered after six hours of natural labor. We were able to take her home after three days. Sarcoidosis was suspected, and a biopsy was performed on the placenta. No sarcoid granulomas were found. The baby was a healthy five pounds, seven ounces, and the delivery was all-natural and without incident. Even after delivery the swelling and lack of circulation, although intermittent, continued. I noticed that the numbness was exacerbated by the cold weather or any overexertion. I mentioned this to the doctor and, of course, his response was to decrease activity. Give me a break! I am the mother of two boys four and two, and a newborn, is he a comedian? I could not afford a housekeeper, and I moved away from any help I would have had in New York. We closed on our home in May, and that sealed my fate. There were seven oak trees in the backyard, and when we viewed the property we were attracted by the size of the yard. It was spring when we moved in, and it looked as though no one had bothered to rake. Little did I know that this was the normal load of leaves after winter, and I was literally knee deep in leaves! Two hundred bags of leaves later, we had half an acre of dirt to reseed if we wanted grass by the summer. You know the old saying, "Buyer beware!" When we first looked at the house, how was I to know, with a baby in my arms, and the yard was covered with leaves? Well, the seller saw us coming. I would rake a pile of leaves, the boys would jump in them, and so on; but it finally got done. I started getting lesions on my hands, but they weren't cuts or bruises. I didn't know what they were. Soon thereafter, I noticed the numbness was particularly unrelieved by medication. Then came one of the worst nights of my life. It was around June 1995. I went to bed and woke up in the wee hours of the morning in pain that I will never forget. It is pain that cannot be described. I jumped up and nearly collapsed to the floor. I let out an incomprehensible sound. My husband turned on the light and looked at my arms, and they were completely gray. My right index finger was completely black, and my hands looked like baseball mitts. There was barely any circulation in my arms or legs. I started shaking my arms and screaming and crying at the same time, "There's no circulation, there's no circulation." I forced my body to stand and started doing this combination—jumping up and down and running in place dance and shaking my arms, and nothing would make the circulation return to my limbs. In desperation, I began to throw my body against the wall over and over and over, banging my limbs in concert while my husband watched in confusion and horror. Finally, the circulation returned. I don't remember how long it took for my circulation to return. All I could do was collapse to the floor and cry uncontrollably. The next morning, which was actually only a few hours later, we were at the emergency room and then off to the office of a rheumatologist. She prescribed what she described as a low-dose steroid called Medrol, which had to be taken over a six-day period. At that point, I would have taken cyanide to prevent the reoccurrence of the events of the night before. Side effect: weight gain. Within two weeks I gained twenty pounds. My daughter was five months old when this incident occurred. When I had given birth to her, I weighed 129 pounds. When I saw the rheumatologist, I weighed in at 130 pounds. She explained that weight gain was just a side effect of the medication. She attributed the "episode" to the disease process of sarcoidosis. She further postulated that Raynaud's phenomenon could also have caused the attack. In other words, she didn't know with any certainty what caused my circulation to stop.

Raynaud's Phenomenon

Raynaud's is a condition that makes it harder for blood to reach certain areas of the body. Blood vessels tighten under the skin and can interrupt blood flow. This occurs with exposure to the cold or when strong emotions trigger blood vessel spasms that interrupt blood flow in the fingers, toes, ears, and nose. Raynaud's may also result from other diseases that affect the blood vessels. Sometimes in severe cases, painful sores may appear on the fingers or toes. When Raynaud's appears by itself, absent of any other medical condition, it is called Raynaud's or primary Raynaud's, and the blood vessels will return to normal afterward. When the disease appears with an autoimmune disease, then it is called Raynaud's phenomenon.

This is an illustration of hands after they have been affected by Raynaud's.

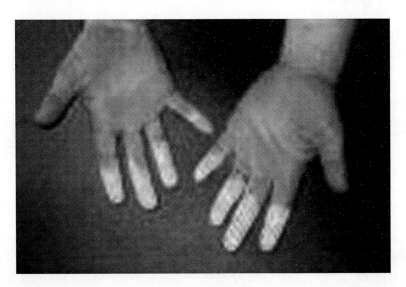

Another incident occurred. It was June and the central air was on. My nickname for my husband is Mr. Freeze when the weather is warm because he keeps the thermostat as low as he possibly can. My husband is 6 feet 5 inches tall built like a linebacker and perspires easily. He keeps the house so cold you can see your breath. We learned quickly about Georgia's summer nights and heat waves. We learned to appreciate the central air as opposed to the window units we had in New York, but with my circulatory problems, the cool air only exacerbated my condition. In the colder months, I maintained a comfort zone of seventy-five degrees, but I would also soon pay for a warm house as well. Interrupted blood flow or Raynaud's can occur without any association to any other symptom of disease; and it is usually associated with lupus, rheumatoid arthritis, or something as simple as repeated typing or playing the piano. These attacks last from minutes to hours. As the mother of a four-year-old, a two-year-old, and a five-month-old, I had my hands full; and I certainly filled the quota for strong emotions triggering the Raynaud's. Her medical opinion regarding my care was to be a continued regimen of steroids, which could lead to serious side effects like Cushing's disease, kidney disease, serious mood swings, and death. In light of the continued weight gain and the fact that the steroids only increased circulation and did not relieve the swelling and pain, we did not see eye to eye, so I sought other medical advice and went on a diet.

I did not have another episode until December 1, 1996, exactly six months after the first. Two days prior to this episode, I noticed swelling and inflammation in the right arm and tingling in the middle right fingers. When the attack occurred, it was limited to the right arm and hand. The loss of feeling, circulation, pain, swelling, and discoloration in the right hand was not relieved; and I immediately went to the emergency room. The doctor noted that the skin on the tips of the index and middle fingers were peeling, and the nail bed of the right index finger was discolored. He further noted that there is an "erythematous hue to the skin of the entire dorsum of the hand." Perhaps that came from my trying to "jump-start" my circulation by slamming my arm against the wall. His diagnosis was vasculitis in the right arm and a referral to a rheumatologist.

My first appointment was with a rheumatologist who was highly recommended by the hospital three days later on December 4, 1996. Upon examination I was advised that my liver was enlarged, although liver function was normal, and this was, in fact, another disease process of sarcoidosis. I advised him of my circulation problems, and he advised me to cut down or stop smoking especially in light of my history of sarcoidosis even though there is no lung involvement. He took the time to explain the effect of nicotine on blood vessels. For the first time, I took a doctor's advice seriously. I was given a drug alternative in light of my adamant refusal to take steroids. A few days later, I was working in my yard doing some light gardening, and noticed that my right arm was going numb and turning colors again. This time the right hand had developed blisters and a rash. It was December 18, 1996, and I was back in this rheumatologist's office. I thought the blisters had come from excessive raking. My layperson's diagnosis was more palatable to me because I was not prepared to hear the doctor's diagnosis that these were vasculitic lesions or perhaps a severe Raynaud's phenomenon in my right hand. The doctor explained that both diagnoses were equally possible. Raynaud's can cause digital finger ulcers due to lack of oxygen to the skin cells.

Vasculitis

The network of blood vessels in the body are referred to as the vascular system. A process called vasculitis occurs when the blood is depleted of oxygen, when there is inflammation of the blood, or when there is destruction of the blood vessel wall. It is not known what causes vasculitis, but the two common features are immune system abnormality and inflammation of the blood vessels. The process may be confined to the skin, or it may involve other organ systems. There is lymphocytic vasculitis whereby lymphoma results. There is granulomatous vasculitus that involves other disease processes. These cells include lymphocytes and occasional giant cells, some of which were found in the biopsy of the right hand digit. Vasculitis of the skin can be seen in lesions, nodules, ulcers, nail-fold telangiectasia (dark-red blotches), and digital gangrene. Once the skin lesions have healed, they usually leave a pronounced postinflammatory hyperpigmentation. This disease causes fever, malaise, and mucous membrane ulcers. It is responsible for causing hematuria, hypertension, abdominal pain, joint pain, iritis, and uveitis. There is no cure for this disease, and once again steroids are the first line of defense. Bed rest, prompt treatment, and monitoring are necessary to prevent mortality and to preserve organ function. Needless to say, I cut down all seven oak trees.

SOUTHERN REGIONAL MEDICAL CENTER
Riverdale, Georgia 30274

cc: Dr.

DEC 1 8 1996

ACCT #: 9633600136

PATIENT NAME: BROWN, STACEY   UNIT #: 0557091

DATE OF TREATMENT: 12/01/96   ROOM #: ER-DIS

ATTENDING PHYSICIAN   M.D.

Patient is a thirty-seven-year-old female with the chief complaint
of right arm pain. States that she has had right arm pain,
swelling and inflamation over the last couple of days. Gets
paresthesias and tingling mostly in her middle fingers. Has noted
some peeling of her skin. Had the same episode about a year ago,
it was felt to be a vasculitic response to either sarcoid or other
inflammatory process. Evaluation otherwise was unremarkable.
States that the pain has come back over the last couple of days.
Complains of peeling skin on her fingers. States that at times her
fingertips look blue.

PAST MEDICAL HISTORY: Otherwise unremarkable.

ALLERGIES: She denies any allergies.

PHYSICAL EXAMINATION: VITAL SIGNS: Temperature 99.9. Pulse 86.
Respirations 16. Blood pressure 139/91. HEENT: Unremarkable.
CHEST: Clear. EXTREMITIES: Examination of the right upper
extremity shows some peeling skin on the tips of the index and
middle fingers. There is some discoloration of the nailbed.
Pulses are 2+. There is no inflammatory processes noted in the
joints. There is slight erythematous hue to the skin of the entire
dorsum of the hand.

ASSESSMENT:
1)   Vasculitis reaction of the right arm.

PLAN:
1)   Patient does not want steroids again.
2)   We will treat her with high-dose
3)   She is to return for increasing pain, fever, discoloration.
4)   She is referred to Dr.   of rhuematology this week.

                              , M.D.

JOB #: 2034   BROWN, STACEY
DD: 12/01/96 MPF   UNIT #: 0557091
DT: 12/04/96 WS2   PAGE 1

EMERGENCY DEPARTMENT REPORT

6F/10

DATE	
DEC 1 8 1996	

Stacey Brown

Raynaud's

Vs Vasculitis.

Wt –
B.P

C.o. - ® Hand swells on & off
~ usage

- ® arm feels less numb
from before.

- No new vasculitic changes

Med: 375 X 2

dE: Wt ↔

BP AL

Wrist: J

Hands: healed lesions
® hand.

No lesions finger tips.

Radial pulses good.

All joints N

A: Raynaud's Vs Vasculitis

No steroid

Arr 6 wks.

| 1-29-97 | Conc. WCB |

Progress

CHAPTER EIGHT

Sarcoidosis

Sarcoidosis is a disease of unknown origin. It is classified as an autoimmune disease. For many years, chronic inflammation has been the cause of many of my medical issues. Granulomas may appear in almost any part of the body, but in the case of sarcoidosis, they are most often found in the skin, eyes, lungs, lymph nodes, and liver, and less often appearing in the spleen, bones, central nervous system, heart, skeletal muscles, and joints. In the majority of cases, the granulomas clear up without treatment; however, the tissue remains scarred. Skin eruptions are frequently caused by the disease, and there is no known cure. When sarcoidosis attacks the lungs, which is most common, it is called pulmonary sarcoidosis; however, the residual scarring is called pulmonary fibrosis and can severely interfere with the ability to breathe. When it attacks the eyes, it is called sarcoid uveitis, as it is in my case. Sarcoid granulomas have been found in the heart, breast, bone marrow, brain, kidneys, liver, eyes, and skin. You have to agree, it is a very unusual disease. It has no known cause and will appear and then disappear.

It is hard to believe, but sarcoid granulomas can appear in the breast. If a doctor is not trained, it will be very easy for them to misdiagnose this disease. The most common course of treatment is steroids, in the most severe cases; however, in most cases of sarcoidosis, the disease will clear up on its own, and no treatment is necessary.

CHAPTER NINE

Carpal Tunnel Syndrome

Carpal tunnel syndrome receives its name from the eight bones in the wrist called carpals that form a tunnel-like structure, as you can see in the following illustration.

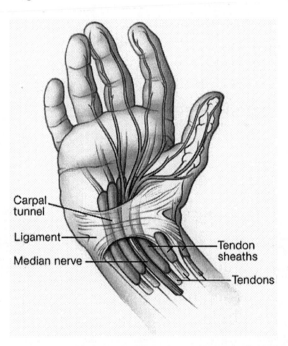

Carpal tunnel
Ligament
Median nerve
Tendon sheaths
Tendons

The structure is filled with flexor tendons that control finger movement and also provide a pathway for the median nerve to reach sensory cells in the hand. Swelling of the tendon sheaths produce what is more commonly referred to as carpal tunnel syndrome. We are in the age of advanced technology, and everything we do requires repeated work with our fingers, making it more likely for us to have

The next two pages are copies of my nerve study, with the names deleted to protect the doctors involved.

Neurological Clinic

Patient:	BROWN,STACEY	Phone:	
Sex:	Female	Physician:	
Age:	41	Test Date:	05/09/01
I.D.#:			
Ref. M.D.:			

History/Comments:

CERVICAL RADICULOPATHY

Motor Nerve Study

Right Median Nerve

Rec Site: APB STIM SITE	Lat (ms)	Norm Lat	Amp (mV)	Norm Amp	C.V. (m/s)	Norm C.V.
Wrist	4.5	2.8-4	7.4	6-16		
Elbow	8.7		6.7	>4	57.6	49-70

Right ULNAR Nerve

Rec Site: ADQ STIM SITE	Lat (ms)	Norm Lat	Amp (mV)	Norm Amp	C.V. (m/s)	Norm C.V.
Wrist	2.7	2-3.4	4.7	4-12		
B.Elbow	5.8		3.8	>5	64.7	49-70
A.Elbow	8.3		3.3	>5	52.0	>42.8

Sensory Nerve Study

Right Radial Nerve

Rec Site: Wrist STIM SITE	Lat (ms)	Norm Lat	Amp (uV)	Norm Amp
Index	2.3	1-3.0	40.3	

Right Ulnar Palmar Nerve

Rec Site: Wrist STIM SITE	Lat (ms)	Norm Lat	Amp (uV)	Norm Amp
Palm	1.6	1.5-2	9.7	>5.0

Right Med Palmar Nerve

Rec Site: Wrist STIM SITE	Lat (ms)	Norm Lat	Amp (uV)	Norm Amp
Palm	2.9	1.5-2	2.0	>8.0

Patient: **BROWN,STACEY**   Test Date: 05/09/01
I.D.#:

F-Wave Study

Right Median Nerve
Rec Site: APB
Stim Site: Wrist

	Latency	Normal
	ns	Latency
F wave	26.17	22-31

Right ULNAR Nerve
Rec Site: ADM
Stim Site: Wrist

	Latency	Normal
	ns	Latency
F wave	26.67	21-32

EMG Study

Name	Ins Act	Fibs	PSW	Fascics	Polyph	MU Amp	MU Dur	Config	Pattern	Int Pat	Recruit
R. Biceps Brachi. Normal	norm	none	none	none	none	norm	norm	norm	norm	full	norm
R. Brachioradialis Normal	norm	none	none	none	none	norm	norm	norm	norm	full	norm
R. Pronator Ter. Normal	norm	none	none	none	none	norm	norm	norm	norm	full	norm
R. Triceps Normal	norm	none	none	none	none	norm	norm	norm	norm	full	norm
R. Abd.Pol.Br.	norm	none	none	none	none	inc	inc	norm	norm	full	norm

Summary/Interpretation:
MODERATE CARPAL TUNNEL PRESENT ON RIGHT.
REFER TO DR.   TO CONSIDER A RELEASE.

carpal tunnel syndrome. The symptoms usually start with pain in the hand and wrist, radiating up the arm accompanied by tingling. As symptoms worsen, there is reduced grip strength, and it will become more difficult to do simple tasks like repeated typing, playing the piano and video games, or grabbing small objects.

In order to determine the existence or severity of carpal tunnel syndrome, the doctor will conduct a sensory nerve study.

Therapy involves a splint, immobilizing the wrist, nonsteroidal drugs, and perhaps, in severe cases, a lidocaine injection into the median nerve to relieve the swelling and pain. However, these measures only provide temporary relief. The majority of patients recover completely. It is only in rare cases that surgical intervention is necessary. In that case, the doctor will go into the wrist and sever the band of tissue around the wrist to reduce the pressure on the median nerve. I opted not to have surgery.

Let's face it. We are not going to stop playing video games, typing, or doing any of the activities that require repeated motion of our fingers and hands. As such we will take anti-inflammatory medication, reduce the repeated motion, or engage in hand-strengthening exercises before we are willing to undergo such a radical procedure. In some rare cases, the loss of circulation is unbearable, and a release is the only option that may be reasonable. The diagram illustrates how the pressure on the median nerve is released; however, there are no guarantees. Life happens. We have to work, and we choose to play. Repeated use is inevitable, and so is recurring carpal tunnel syndrome.

CHAPTER TEN

Faith

We joined a local church soon after moving to Georgia, and I was ready to give up my ugly and smelly habit of cigarette smoking. My blood vessels would be happy too. My new rheumatologist had led this patient to water, and now I was ready to drink. He explained that smoking was only exacerbating the attacks of Raynaud's and vasculitis. When I joined this church in or around November of 1998, I had no idea that on New Year's Eve a miracle would take place. My family and I were there for our first New Year's service, and as they say in deliverance worship, "the church was on fire." We were singing, dancing, shouting, and praising the Lord. Our pastor asked if anyone needed to be healed. I began to walk to the front of the church and stood on line. I was thinking to myself, *I can't wait to get out of here and break open that bottle of champagne.* I was just walking slowly and following the others, not realizing that the line had moved so quickly, and I was standing right in front of my pastor. Now it is easy to explain that he could smell the cigarettes on my clothes, but to this day I can only explain it away as divine intervention when he shouted *liquor* as he touched my body because I was not a regular drinker. I would drink on holidays or while on vacation. After all, it was New Year's Eve, and it was time to break out the bubbly. I was *so* embarrassed. He grabbed the top of my head and started praying, speaking in tongues, and calling on Jesus. Suddenly it felt as though I was a cigarette and someone had lit a match underneath my feet. My body began to shake, and his voice began to fade. All I remember when I came to was the voices of the choir and the missionaries and church mothers standing around me to protect me from the crowd. They helped me to my feet, and I couldn't stand straight. I felt as though I were drunk. My pastor would not leave me alone. He explained that I was drunk with the Holy Spirit. He had the biggest smile on his face. I couldn't help but smile and be happy too. I couldn't walk straight. I was literally walking like a drunk and felt like I was drunk, but it was different. The only thing holding me up was the wall. I didn't know whether to laugh or cry, so I did both. I started praising God as though I had lost my mind. I will never forget that day as long as I live. I never touched another cigarette or drink since. Christ literally knocked the taste out of my mouth.

I started smoking when I was sixteen—just a puff, not inhaling—because my friends were doing it. I began to inhale at seventeen and started buying by the pack by the time I reached eighteen and had reached a twenty-year one-and-a-half-pack-to-two packs-a-day habit that was broken in minutes without the aid of drugs or hypnosis. All I needed was God and the power of Christ. In his word he promised that he would never leave me or forsake me. He has always kept his word. We have to remember to put our faith in God and not in man (Psalm 118:8). It is the power and wisdom of the word of God that gets us through each day and each crisis in our lives. I had to remember this in order to stay focused.

The lungs on the left are smoker's lungs, and the lungs on the right are healthy lungs. The difference is so apparent. Bless God for saving and changing me.

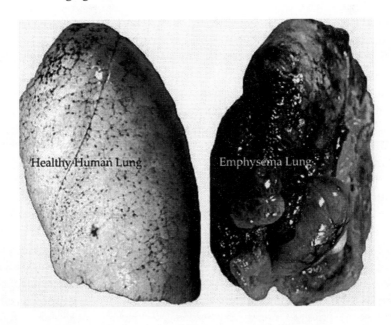

Healthy Human Lung   Emphysema Lung

With each new diagnosis, I never lost my faith in God. There were times when I had to go to the doctor five times out of a seven-day week. I was exhausted emotionally and financially.

After I stopped smoking, the vasculitis attacks ceased. Hindsight allows me to see that if I did not stop smoking that New Year's Eve, one of the several surgeries that followed that night may have been accompanied with complications, or one of them may have been my last.

CHAPTER ELEVEN

Tonsillitis

In or around August 1999, I began to have trouble with my throat. Not just minor sore throat irritation, but raw, cutting discomfort accompanied by a fever of 102 degrees or greater, a can't—swallow type of irritation. I went to see an ear, nose, and throat specialist. She was wonderful and extremely knowledgeable. She advised me to gargle with undiluted hydrogen peroxide as part of my daily regimen. However, in spite of diligently following her instructions and repeated ingestion of antibiotics, my throat would flare up once a month for approximately six months like clockwork. It seemed that each bout was getting worse than the last, and the fevers were getting higher until they peaked at 104 and held on. Finally, every course of treatment failed, I was scheduled for surgery January 13, 2000, at Northside Hospital.

I thought tonsillectomies were for children. I found out firsthand that I was wrong. The tonsil is what we see when we open our mouths and look into the back of the throat. It is part of the body's immune system by filtering out germs that come into the body through the mouth and nose. As bacteria enters the body, it can become infected and results in the tonsils and adenoids swelling. Adenoids are not visible when you first open your mouth because they are high in the throat behind the nose and the roof of the mouth, but they can be seen with the assistance of special instruments. The tonsils are a mass of visible tissue hanging down and around the throat or the walls of the pharynx, which form a lymphoid tissue ring consisting of cells similar to the lymphocytes in the bloodstream. These are special cells that function to fight disease. These lymphoid cells are like a giant sponge and absorb or digest bacteria or other foreign bodies by phagocytes, and the process is called phagocytosis. When this condition occurs, the lymphoid cells protect the pharynx from invasion by disease-producing bacteria, and the tonsils become infected. This condition is called tonsillitis. At the main site of infection the tonsils swell, become red and inflamed, and show a surface coating of white spots. Acute cases of tonsillitis frequently form pus and are treated with antibiotics. Acute, chronic, recurrent tonsillitis is treated by surgical removal called tonsillectomy. Recovery is usually a few weeks and is accompanied by a very sore throat.

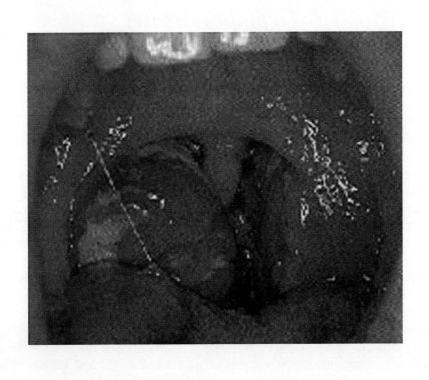

CHAPTER TWELVE

The National Commission on Orphan Diseases

In the 1980s, Congress sanctioned a study; and it was concluded that 31 percent of persons with rare disorders took between one and five years to obtain a proper diagnosis, 15 percent went six years or more without a diagnosis, 45 percent reported extreme financial hardship to them and their families, and 42 percent reported that the illness kept them from working or attending school. The primary objective is to raise awareness. There are an alarming number of health professionals who are not familiar with these diseases, and these patients suffer needlessly physically, emotionally, and financially. The report was released to Congress in 1989. Once diagnosed, 76 percent of these patients reported they could not find any information about the disease. As a result the National Organization for Rare Disorders, or NORD, was established in 1983. They are committed to working toward the prevention, treatment, and cure of rare orphan diseases. It is a wonderful organization that not only provides information about the particular disease, but they will also provide prescription drugs to people who cannot afford them. NORD honors companies that have developed products to treat serious diseases. One such company developed a drug for treatment of chronic noninfectious uveitis. As you may recall, this is one of the diseases I suffer with. If you have a rare disorder, it probably can be found in the Index of Rare Diseases. NORD has a rare disease database that covers more than 1,150 diseases.

NORD now offers free physicians' guides to rare diseases, and it also provides medication-assistance programs, which provides drugs to those patients who cannot afford them. If you buy flowers for any occasion from NORD's From You Flowers Inc., 20 percent of the purchase price will be donated to NORD research. NORD is a wonderful association that provides charitable long-distance medical air travel assistance. For those who just want to read about rare diseases or those affected by it, the NORD Resource Guide is now available in libraries.

While in the waiting room of my oncologist/hematologist, I heard one horror story after another. In my case, the doctor's lack of knowledge only delayed my treatment; but in these patients' cases, it costs them their lives. For two years, I was under the care of one neurologist, who never heard of the rare disease that I have before I was referred to another, who properly diagnosed my condition immediately.

The jurisdictional cap on medical malpractice in Georgia is not equal to the value of a life and certainly will not bring them back. This is another reason I decided to write this book. Not only because I have so many rare diseases, but because I feel I can be a voice for many. Advocacy has to begin somewhere, and let it begin at home. The medical community at large has to take responsibility and begin to at least minimally familiarize themselves with orphan diseases. If doctors run into a situation that they are unfamiliar with, they should utter these words to their patient, "I don't know what's wrong with you!" Quite often, the treating physician will not release the patient from his or her care because they will not admit that they do not know what is wrong. I believe in testing to rule out a particular disease. However, when a physician tells the patient he or she has a cold and sends him or her home and it is in fact emphysema or lung cancer and fails to listen to the patient, then that is unforgivable. In my case, I continually complained of neck pain, and in the physician's notes he wrote, "pain switches," which indicated he thought I was faking. It's a shame because this "doctor" is a licensed neurologist and psychologist who could not admit to me that he never heard of the rare disease even after I told him of the diagnosis. I sought a second opinion and discovered that I have a serious, rare degenerative disease of the spine, along with **cord compression**. How do you fake cord compression? As I indicated earlier, radiology reports do not lie. Soon after this encounter, I was diagnosed with multiple sclerosis; and then every month, like clockwork, it seemed I was diagnosed with one autoimmune disease after another! The cost is too high! What is the measure of accountability?

America is the greatest country in the world; and with our modern technology and methods of detection, a simple blood draw should be able to detect the presence of diseases in the human body, including orphan diseases. If we haven't done it, then Congress should be sanctioned to fund a study to have it done. It will save time, lives, and money. We are the richest country in the world with the poorest and most underfunded health care policies. Our elderly and poor should be treated with care and respect, yet they are treated as an annoyance. The poor use the emergency room as their personal doctor's office because they cannot afford health care. The middle class can afford a health care policy but cannot afford the co-pay. We have a problem, America! We have to change the face of health care.

CHAPTER THIRTEEN

Tietze's Syndrome/Costochondritis

I had been complaining of chest pain just above the heart for as long as I could remember, but my complaints went unheeded. The lump is palpable, raised, hard to the touch, very sore, and very painful. My repeated complaints of a "chest wall mass" had been finally diagnosed. It was not until I went to my primary care physician and asked for a second opinion. He ordered an MRI and referred me to a local surgeon. She took one look at the film and told me

The following is an illustration of Tietze's syndrome or costochondritis.

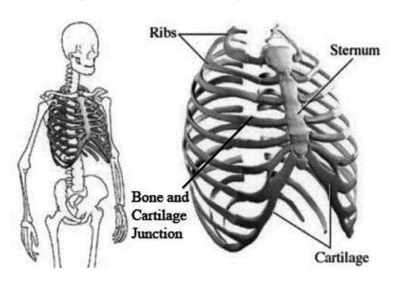

I had a rare condition called Tietze's syndrome, also known as costochondritis or chondropathia tuberosa, for which there is no cure. Here we are again, the fourth receptor of prostaglandins rearing its ugly head. The cause of the disease is unknown. For those familiar with this rare disease, it is easily recognizable once the patient complains of pain, swelling, and tenderness in a localized area. It is palpable in a spindle shape or fusiform (spindle shape and tapering at each end), and swelling may occur in one or more of the four upper ribs. The onset of pain is gradual, accompanied with a sensation that is dull or sharp, mild or severe, gripping or neuralgic in nature. The condition is easily confirmed with an x-ray or MRI of the chest wall. Sudden coughing or deep breathing accentuates the pain and is often followed by swelling. Tietze's syndrome is like having a fractured rib that never heals. The treatment consists of localized heat to reduce nerve root irritation and anti-inflammatory drugs or pain medication and rest.

Just above my left breast there is a sore spindle-shaped mass that never heals. It is raised, hard to the touch, and it is located between the costochondral junction and the second and fifth costal ribs. The pain can occur at the junction of the bony and cartilaginous part of the ribs. What makes this disease so dangerous is that it mimics the symptoms of a heart attack and bone cancer, and the pain is easily aggravated with deep breathing, sneezing, or twisting motions.

CHAPTER FOURTEEN

Cervical Myofascial Pain Syndrome

Cervical myofascial pain syndrome is a painful musculoskeletal condition and is a common cause of musculoskeletal pain. It is characterized by the development of trigger points. A trigger point—or a sensitive, painful area in the muscle—may develop due to a number of causes. These factors can cause trigger points: sudden trauma to musculoskeletal tissues, injury to intervertebral discs, chronic fatigue syndrome, repetitive motions, excessive exercise, muscle strain due to overactivity or lack of activity, nutritional deficiencies, hormonal changes, nervous tension, stress, or chilling of areas of the body. The fascia is a tough connective tissue, which spreads throughout the body in a three-dimensional web from head to foot without interruption, and it surrounds every muscle, bone, nerve, blood vessel, and organ of the body all the way down to the cellular level. Therefore, any malfunction of the fascial system due to trauma, poor posture, or inflammation can result in abnormal pressure on the nerves, muscles, bones, or organs. The result is pain throughout the body. Trigger points produce localized pain, although the trigger points of MPS generally involve the body as a whole. Medical evidence, however, such as x-rays, MRIs, myleograms, CAT scans do not show the fascia. These trigger points can be seen upon examination by a trained eye. A trigger point is a hyperirritable area located in a palpable taut band of muscle fibers; in other words, the doctor can feel an area that is like a tight band of muscle. In some severe cases, the taut band is raised and can be plainly seen. The most common trigger points are the trapezius, the levator scapulae, rhomboids, supraspinatus, and infraspinatus. The trapezius muscle is a very large but thin muscle located between the shoulder blade and the neck. The levator scapulae are the muscles that allow our head to rotate left and right, up and down. Rhomboids are located below the levator scapulae muscles. The first sets are called minor rhomboids, and the next sets are called major rhomboids. They are responsible for holding the scapula against the thoracic wall. The supraspinatus and infraspinatus or rotator cuff muscles are the second most common injuries. One of the most common symptoms is dizziness. Patients often exhibit poor posture, rounded shoulders, and protracted scapulae. However, any trauma can exacerbate this condition: a car accident, intense cold due to the weather or excessive air conditioning. Chronic infections, nutritional deficiencies, stress, or poor posture at the workplace can cause cervical myofascial syndrome. Fibromyalgia, on the other hand, is a much more serious disease, although the disorders are related. It is the rheumatic hardening of the muscle, and there are a specific number of trigger points for each condition.

<u>NEUROLOGICAL CLINIC</u>

BROWN, STACEY   03/28/01

<u>SUBJECTIVE</u>: This 41-year-old African-American female is seen in followup. She is on 10 mg t.i.d., and is having good relief of her neck pain. ·

Her MRI Study showed a mild degree of spondylosis at C5-6, C6-7. She did not have any nerve root compression noted.

<u>OBJECTIVE:</u> On examination, the blood pressure is 120/88. Her examination is otherwise unchanged.

<u>IMPRESSION</u>:   1. Cervical myofascial pain syndrome.

<u>PLAN:</u>
1. Continue
2. Follow-up visit here in one month's time.

_____
us, M.D., Ph.D.

CHAPTER FIFTEEN

Chronic Degenerative Disc Disease: Genetic Breakdown

Degenerative changes in the spine and those that usually cause loss of structure or loss of function usually occur with age. This process affects the intervertebral discs, and it is a known fact that it is a gradual process. Wear and tear would be the natural process to break down the intervertebral disc over time—approximately ten to twenty years. The term *degenerative disc disease* means that one or more of your discs has sustained injury and the ability of the spine to absorb stress has diminished. The annulus is the first portion of the disc that seems to be injured. The annulus is the outer ring of tough ligament material that holds vertebrae together. If there is rapid loss of water content, desiccation, the disc will lose its ability to act as a cushion and dry up, leading to stress, tears, space narrowing, and the spine will shift; and this process will repeat itself. Because of the pressure, bone spurs called osteophytes will form around the disc spaces. This is the body's response to try to stop the excess motion of the spine, and, of course, it repeats itself. Then the bone spurs start to grow into the spinal canal and press on the spinal cord and nerves. This condition is called spinal stenosis. From here, pain can be felt in the buttocks and shoulders. Pain can be so great it can be as though you are experiencing a heart attack. Remember, it is the loss of cartilage in one or more joints. However, there are other changes that will affect the normal structure of the spine. Osteoarthritis is named the number 1 factor in women over fifty-five. I had onset at approximately age forty-one. The question is, what caused the fast forward button to be pushed in my body? Primary osteoarthritis is related to aging. While there are millions of children and young adults who experience some form of arthritis, there isn't any single known cause of osteoarthritis; however, there are several risk factors. Usually repetitive use of joints causing pain and swelling or desiccation of discs in the spine is the primary cause of osteoarthritis. However, I had onset at age forty-one of degenerative osteoarthritis in the hands. Medically, I am too young, for there to have been such a degree of deterioration of degenerative osteoarthritis in the spine at such a rapid pace. So let's look at other factors. My medical records will show that I already had arthritis in the hands, and for that reason I was prescribed Vioxx and Celebrex at the age of forty-two for a period that exceeds, give or take, six months. Prior to January 1999, I had **no** problems whatsoever, and medical records will reflect there was no substantial injury to, or anything wrong with, my back insofar as degenerative disc disease is concerned.

The prostaglandin receptor that affects calcium movement, in this case, is essential for building strong **bones**. Then a drug is introduced, and a deficit can affect bone formation. So can this explain what happened when my body suddenly developed all of these rare diseases for which there is no explanation or genetic predisposition? My condition was exacerbated, and a process that would have taken **twenty** years occurred within a period of **three** years. The medical records will show the facts as follows.

The winter months passed slowly after my recovery from brain surgery. The cold weather was wreaking havoc on my bones because of the osteoarthritis. The pressure in my neck and pain in the left shoulder area was worsening. I was fighting migraines in an almost-daily basis. I was having trouble sleeping because of leg pain, and it felt as though I couldn't rest comfortably because my neck could never be positioned properly or there was always too much pressure on my hips. I was miserable. I conveyed these feelings to my doctor, and he started me on several drugs to control the migraines until I finally settled on one. Then one night, the temperature dropped to thirty-two degrees. The heat was on, but my husband woke up in the middle of the night with the pillows soaked with perspiration. Instead of taking off the covers or turning the heat down, he got up and opened the window a crack over our bed. The cold air sent me straight to the emergency room. The pain radiated straight down my spine. The cold sailed through my body, and, as my children described it, I flapped on the floor like a fish out of water. I couldn't get up. I was cold, stiff, sore, and in so much pain. I didn't know whether to cry or scream. After arriving at the emergency room, a soft cervical collar was placed on my neck.

As a point of reference, starting with a period immediately following the surgery for removal of the cervical posterior mass, the spine showed good alignment, and the intervertebral disc spaces were well maintained as of October 31, 2000. However it did not take long for my circumstances to change.

In less than a year later, although disc height is maintained, there is loss of signal from C3-C7 with spurring, together with small focal disc bulge and mild degenerative desiccation and spondylitic changes. From October 31, 2000, to April 22, 2002, this MRI showed loss of disc height, disc protrusion, cord compression, spondylosis, extruded herniation, cord flattening, and nerve root irritation. There is evidence of degenerative disc disease affecting the cervical, thoracic, and lumbar spine. This disease is common to those over forty; however, what is not common is that the whole spine is affected, the age of onset, and the rapid deterioration.

Examples of Disc Problems

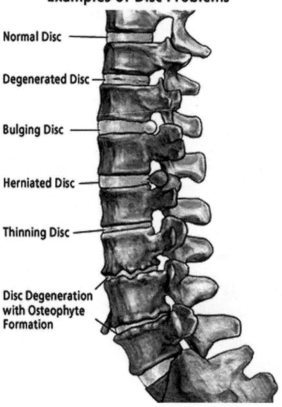

Normal Disc

Degenerated Disc

Bulging Disc

Herniated Disc

Thinning Disc

Disc Degeneration
with Osteophyte
Formation

p.o

PIEDMONT HOSPITAL

DUPLICATE   FINAL

Name: BROWN,STACEY PRICE
DOB: 05/23/59   Age: 41Y   Sex: F
Ordered Date/Time:
Ck-In Date/Time: 10/31/00 1134

Location: DIS - ODC
MR# P002124569
Acct#: P0030590396

Deliver to:

Attend. Dr:
Admit. Dr:
Ref. Dr:
Ord.
PCP:

Chk-in #	Exam	Desc	Ord. Diag.
654187	70115	CR SPINE CERVICAL AP & LATERAL	V72.83-OTH SPCF PREOP EXAM

AP and lateral views of the cervical spine were performed. The
prevertebral soft tissues are within normal limits. There is good
alignment of the cervical vertebral bodies. The intervertebral disc
spaces are well maintained. There is no evidence of acute fracture or
subluxation.

IMPRESSION: No evidence of acute fracture or subluxation.

Read By: JOI
sed By: MD
Time Released: 10/31/00 1651

SW
10/31/00 1651

FINAL   Radiology Report

XXXXXXFINALXXXXXFINALXXXXXXXFINALREPORTXXXXXXFINALXXXFINALXXXXXXXXXXXXXXXXXXX

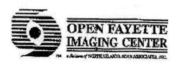

OPEN FAYETTE IMAGING CENTER
a division of NORTH ATLANTA SCAN ASSOCIATES, INC.

Brown,Stacey

DOB:05/23/59

MD

Date of Exam:03/14/01

214

MRI CERVICAL SPINE WITH AND WITHOUT CONTRAST

HISTORY: This is a 41 year old female with previous neck surgery and neck pain radiating down to the left shoulder.

DESCRIPTION: Sagittal T1 and T2 weighted images are performed from the mid-brainstem through the T2 vertebra. Axial static T1 and T2 weighted images were performed from the C3 to the T1 level. Following the administration of Magnevist contrast, axial and sagittal T1 weighted images were repeated.

FINDINGS: Mild straightening of the cervical spine is noted consistent with cervical paraspinal muscle spasm. A signal from within the cervical vertebral bodies is unremarkable. The disc height is overall fairly well maintained. There is mild loss of T2 signal from within the C3-C4, C4-C5, C5-C6, and C6-C7 discs consistent with mild degenerative desiccation of these discs.

With attention to the individually imaged cervical discs, the C2-C3 disc appears normal. At C3-C4 there is mild loss of disc signal associated with a few very tiny posterior spurs. At C4-C5 there is a fairly large right posterior paracentral spondylitic spur noted which abuts but which does not clearly compress the cervical spinal cord. The C5-C6 level demonstrates a small focal subligamentous disc bulge, without frank disc herniation. This does not compress the cervical spinal cord. The neural foramina are normal bilaterally. The C6-C7 disc again shows some very minimal spondylitic changes posteriorly. The neural foramina are widely patent. No compression of the exiting nerve roots is noted.

The cervical spinal cord appears normal throughout its course. No areas of abnormal signal are noted from within the cord.

The extra-axial soft tissues are unremarkable. No discrete masses are identified.

Following the administration of Magnevist contrast, no significant abnormal enhancement is seen.

IMPRESSION: Mildly abnormal cervical MRI study demonstrating:
1.   Posterior spondylitic spurring at C3-C4 and C4-C5 levels without clear-cut compression of the cervical spinal cord or exiting nerve roots.

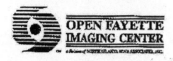

OPEN FAYETTE IMAGING CENTER
a division of NORTH ATLANTA SCAN ASSOCIATES, INC.

Brown,Stacey

Date of Exam:03/14/01

continued...

MRI CERVICAL SPINE WITH AND WITHOUT CONTRAST

IMPRESSION (Continued)

2.   Mild degenerative desiccation is noted of the C3-C4 to C5-C6 discs.
3.   No frank disc herniation or nerve root compression is noted. No soft tissue masses are seen.

MD

as/April 5, 2001/

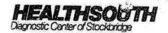

HEALTHSOUTH
Diagnostic Center of Stockbridge

Account #: 030232   fax report
Film Jacket #: 00030232
Name: BROWN. STACY
Date of Birth: 5/23/59 Sex: F
Ref: 00116   I M.D.
Date of Procedure: 4/22/02

EXAM: MRI OF THE CERVICAL SPINE

INDICATION: 42-year-old female with neck pain radiating to the left upper extremity.

TECHNIQUE: Views of the cervical spine were performed with axial images from C2 through T1.

FINDINGS: Alignment and bony integrity are normal.

Cranial-cervical junction and C2-3 are normal.

At the C3-4 level, there is minimal degenerative change with tiny central discal protrusion on axial #5/24, none of which exert any significant compressive effect.

The C4-5 level is mildly degenerate with bulging and minor uncovertebral osteophyte formation without significant neural compressive effect. As noted on axial #8/24, right paracentral disc causes mild right-sided cord indentation and may give rise to some discogenic pain.

The C5-6 level is decreased in height and mildly spondylitic, although the foramina appear patent on 11/24. A right paracentral HNP impinges slightly on the cord, but without significantly compressing it.

The C6-7 level is degenerate with loss of disc height. As seen best on T1-weighted #5/9, extruded disc extends both above and below the level of the disc space and as seen on axial #12/20, the HNP extends off primarily to the left compressing the left cord slightly and also causing left C7 nerve root irritation. No significant spondylosis is seen at this time at this level.

The C7-T1 and lower levels are normal. The cord, although impinged upon multiply and particularly at the C6-7 level, does not show signs of myelomalacia. Although he C6-7 level appears to be the most prominent left-sided abnormality, left-sided spondylosis at the C5-6 level does cause some indentation of the left ventral lateral recess and may be a contributing factor to the left-sided pain.

Continued

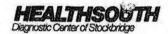

HEALTHSOUTH
Diagnostic Center of Stockbridge

STACY BROWN #30232
APRIL 22, 2002
PAGE 2

IMPRESSION: Degenerative disc disease with mild spondylosis from C3 to C6 without significant neural compressive effect, but with cord impingement or indentation at each level of relatively minor degree.

C6-7: Left paracentral superiorly and inferiorly extruded herniation with left-sided cord flattening and left C7 nerve root irritation.

DGS/vlo
Transcribed: 4/23/02

DANIEL G.   , M.D.

In an attempt to "fix" the problem, my doctor ordered a discogram. It certainly did not sound like a party for my spine, so I asked him to explain the procedure to me before I consented to it. To put it simply, large needles would be placed in my cervical spine at each level from C3 to C6. I would then let the radiologist know when it hurt. If the pain were more intense at one level as opposed to another, then he would want to remove that particular disc. He said that he could not determine from the MRI which disc was causing my problems. He did not mince his words; he said the procedure would be painful and that afterward, pins and needles would be placed in my neck. I respectfully declined and told him I did not wish to be the bride of Frankenstein. Hindsight is always 20/20.

On March 27, 2003, cord compression is now complete, the discs are bulging out of the back of my neck at every level from C3-C7, and my dural sac is now involved together with nerve root sleeves and osteophyte formations. The neurologist I was referred to ordered a myelogram and a CT of my spine. He diagnosed me with a rare disease of the spine, which is discussed later in this book together with degenerative disc disease, mild scoliosis, cord compression, and a host of other problems. All these findings are prior to October 10, 2003—**less than three years!** The radiology reports follow:

PIEDMONT HOSPITAL

DUPLICATE   FINAL

Name: BROWN,STACEY PRICE
DOB: 05/23/59   Age: 43Y   Sex: F
Ordered Date/Time:
Ck-In Date/Time: 03/27/03 0928

Deliver to:

Location: DIS - ODC
MR#   P002124569
Acct#: P0307000251

Attend. Dr:
Admit. Dr:
Ref. Dr:
Ord. Dr.:
PCP: K

Chk-in # Exam   Desc   Ord. Diag.
1307044   74111 CT CERVICAL SPINE WITH   722.0-CERVICAL DISC DISPLAC

There is asymmetric bulging of the disc n the right at C3-C4 with
compression of the dural sac ventrally. This may be touching the
anterior aspect of the cord on the right, but no cord flattening or
deformation is identified. No nerve root sheath compression or
foraminal stenosis is seen.

There appears to be some thickening with possible calcification in the
posterior longitudinal ligament behind the vertebral bodies, starting at
C3 and extending inferiorly. There is compression of the dural sac
ventrally. There may be some compression of the cervical spinal cord
with flattening of the ventral aspect of the cord on the right, behind
the C3 vertebra.

At C4-C5, this may continue or there may be asymmetric bulging of the
disc on the right with cord compression on the right side, possibly
associated with some posterior osteophyte formation. There is
flattening of the ventral aspect of the cord on the right but no
definite compression of the nerve root sleeves is seen.

There is thickening of the longitudinal ligament with calcification on
the right behind the L4 vertebral body, causing compression of the dural
sac. This is touching the anterior aspect of the cord longitudinally on
the right at L4.

At C5-C6, there is an asymmetric extradural defect on the right which is
soft tissue in nature, possibly associated with some posterior

FINAL   CONTINUED   Radiology Report

XXXXXXFINALXXXXXFINALXXXXXXXFINALREPORTXXXXXXFINALXXXFINALXXXXXXXXXXXXXXXXXXXX

PIEDMONT HOSPITAL   Page 2

DUPLICATE   FINAL

Name: BROWN,STACEY PRICE   Location: DIS - ODC
DOB: 05/23/59   Age: 43Y Sex: F   MR#   P002124569
Ordered Date/Time: Acct#: P0307000251
Ck-In Date/Time: 03/27/03 0928

Deliver to: Attend. Dr:
                                        Admit. Dr:
                                        Ref. Dr:
                                        Ord. Dr.:
                                        PCP:

Checkin-Exam Code Summary
1307044-74111

osteophyte formation. Whether this is due to thickening of the
posterior longitudinal ligament or asymmetric focal bulging of the disc,
is not known with absolute certainty. Again, there appears to be some
compression of the ventral aspect of the cord on the right side, which
is mild. No compression of the nerve root sleeves is noted.

At C5 there is again some thickening of the longitudinal ligament
posteriorly with calcification. This is causing some compression of the
dural sac ventrally on the right and may be compressing the right side
of the cord slightly behind the C5 vertebral body.

At C5-C6, there is asymmetric focal bulging of the disc or soft tissue
structures posteriorly on the right side with cord compression on the
right. No nerve root sheath compression is noted. There is only minimal
soft tissue thickening behind the C7 vertebral body. No extradural
defect is noted at C7-T1.

No nerve root sheath compression is seen at C7-T1.

IMPRESSION:

This is a very unusual appearance with soft tissue thickening which
appears to be oriented in longitudinal fashion behind the disc spaces
and vertebral bodies, extending from C3 down to C7. This may represent
some thickening in the posterior longitudinal ligament, some of which is
associated with some calcification. There is compression of the dural
sac ventrally on the right side. There is compression of the cord

FINAL   CONTINUED   Radiology Report

XXXXXXFINALXXXXXFINALXXXXXXXFINALREPORTXXXXXXFINALXXXPINALXXXXXXXXXXXXXXXXXX

DUPLICATE   FINAL

Name: BROWN,STACEY PRICE
DOB: 05/23/59   Age: 43Y Sex: F
Ordered Date/Time:
Ck-In Date/Time: 03/27/03 0928

Location: DIS - ODC
MR#   P002124569
Acct#: P0307000251

Deliver to:

Attend. Dr   L
Admit. Dr: L
Ref. Dr:
Ord. Dr.:
PCP:

Checkin-Exam Code Summary
1307044-74111

longitudinally on the right side. I cannot exclude the possibility of
asymmetric bulging discs at C3-C4, C4-C5, C5-C6 and C6-C7, causing
compression of the cervical spinal cord on the right at these levels,
but this may all be part of a process involving the posterior
longitudinal ligament with thickening of the ligament and compression of
the cord on the right. Clinical correlation is suggested. No nerve
root sheath compression is seen.

                       Read By:
                       Released :
                       Date/Time Released: 03/27/03 1803

KB
03/27/03 1803

PIEDMONT HOSPITAL

Name: BROWN,STACEY PRICE
DOB: 05/23/59 Age: 43Y Sex: F
Ordered Date/Time:
Ck-In Date/Time: 03/27/03 0748

Deliver to: (

Location: DIS - ODC
MR#   P002124569
Acct#: P0307000251

Attend. Dr:
Admit. Dr:
Ref. Dr:
Ord. Dr.:
PCP:

Chk-In # Exam   Desc   Ord. Diag.
1306878 75003 MYELOGRAM CERVICAL*   722.0-CERVICAL DISC DISPLAC

A lumbar puncture was performed in the usual fashion and a myelogram was
performed using Omnipaque 300, injected intrathecally. Contrast was
positioned in the cervical region. No nerve root sheath defects are
identified on the oblique images. No definite cord widening or
compression is noted. ON the swimmer's view, there are double densities
ventrally from C3 down to C7 of uncertain significance. This is not as
well seen on the true lateral view. The cord does not show any definite
evidence of compression, however. A CT scan is pending for further
evaluation of these findings.

IMPRESSION:

No nerve root sheath compression defects are identified. There is some
very minimal scoliosis in the cervicothoracic region. In the swimmer's
view there are some double densities seen from C3 to C7 at multiple
levels which may represent some bulging discs or possibly some
thickening of the ligament flavum. CT is pending for further evaluation
of this finding.

Read By:
Released
Date/Time Released: 03/27/03 1742

KB
03/27/03 1742

FINAL   Radiology Report

XXXXXXFINALXXXXXFINALXXXXXXXFINALREPORTXXXXXXFINALXXXFINALXXXXXXXXXXXXXXXXXXX

PIEDMONT HOSPITAL

DUPLICATE   FINAL

Name: BROWN,STACEY PRICE
DOB: 05/23/59   Age: 44Y   Sex: F
Ordered Date/Time:
Ck-In Date/Time: 03/10/04 1650

Location: DIS - ODC
MR#   P002124569
Acct#: P0407000968

Deliver to

AD

ATLANTA   GA   30309

Attend. Dr:
Admit. Dr:
Ref. Dr:
Ord. Dr.: |
PCP: JONES,KEI

Chk-in # Exam   Desc   Ord. Diag.
1604313 78085   MRI CERVICAL SPINE W/WO   723.1-CERVICALGIA

TECHNIQUE: Sagittal T1 postcontrast, T2 sagittal, axial oblique
gradient echo, sagittal FLAIR and sagittal T1 sequences. No previous
films are available for comparison.

The vertebral bodies have a normal height, alignment and signal
intensity. There is loss of signal at every disc space compatible with
degenerative disc disease. Loss of height at C6-C7. At the C6-C7
level, there is a ventral extradural defect compressing the ventral
thecal sac and the spinal cord. This is to the right of midline. There
is a smaller central defect at C5-C6 with ventral thecal sac
compression. A right paramedian defect is also noted at C4-C5 with
thecal sac and cord compression. The spinal cord has normal signal
intensity and the foramen magnum is normal.

IMPRESSION:

Ventral defect at C4-C5, C5-C6 and C6-C7. Cord compression at C4-C5 and
C6-C7 is noted.

                         Read By:
                         Released $ MD
                         Date/Time   11/04 1544

ME
03/11/04 0845

FINAL   Radiology Report
XXXXXXFINALXXXXXFINALXXXXXXXFINALREPORTXXXXXXFINALXXXFINALXXXXXXXXXXXXXXXXXX

CHAPTER SIXTEEN

Cervical Spondylosis

The MRI of April 22, 2002, noted mild spondylosis. Spondylosis is a degenerative intervertebral disc disease with secondary osteoarthritis. Structural changes from degeneration and compression change disc height. As the disease progresses, there is nerve root compression and narrowing of the spinal canal. The spinal canal contains the nerves that are responsible for communication with the rest of the body. Compression of the spinal canal leads to wasting, diminished reflexes, loss of anterior horn cells, and disruption of ascending and descending sensory and motor pathways. The results are **chronic pain**, gait disturbance, and bladder complaints. Hello, adult diapers!

There are many diseases associated with cervical spondylosis. The disease will cause pain in the neck, lower back, legs, and arms. It is also responsible for muscle weakness, arm weakness, and difficulty of movement. The lumbar region will also be stiff as a result of this disease. As disc degeneration occurs, stresses result along the ventral aspect of the spinal canal, and bone spurs may begin to form. If the bone spurs are serious enough, they may interfere with your ability to swallow. In my case, the spurring has already begun to interfere with my ability to swallow, and I was advised that surgical intervention would be too risky at this point. Neck and shoulder pain result in occipital headache, and degenerative changes in the facet joints are common. When I move, you can hear popping in the neck and joints as a result of this disease. The joint popping is quite audible. As a result, there is nerve-root irritation in the neck, which can sometimes be relieved with a soft cervical collar, pain medication, and rest. Bone spurs appeared on my MRIs as osteophytes and reveals the extent of damage to the cervical spine. Although diseases associated with degenerative changes are common, their rapid progression is not, as in my case. Bone spurs cause nerve-root compression. Although rest, medication, and therapy are recommended, there is no cure for the chronic pain, and, ultimately, decompression of the spine may be recommended to provide relief.

Please note the radiology report was dated July 21, 2003, which is again less than the projected three years. There is mild cervical spondylosis and anterior spurring. Two years later, in the radiology report dated April 21, 2005, spondylosis has now become multilevel, and left facet arthropathy is predominant on the left side. It can be traced from levels C7 through T1. Left facet arthropathy is a condition whereby disease progression has led to **impaired deep pain perception; disease progression causes severe pain, bone overgrowth, coarse or grating audible crepitus sounds, and deformity.** My children laugh at me when I attempt to dance or when I move because you can actually hear my bones creak and crack, but in reality it is not funny. When I hug someone or they hug me, I literally crack. This is certainly evidence of calcium movement and absorption in the body in the body being affected—the seventh receptor of prostaglandins. There is also evidence of canal stenosis. Please note that all this occurred within a period of less than two years as evidenced by the radiology reports.

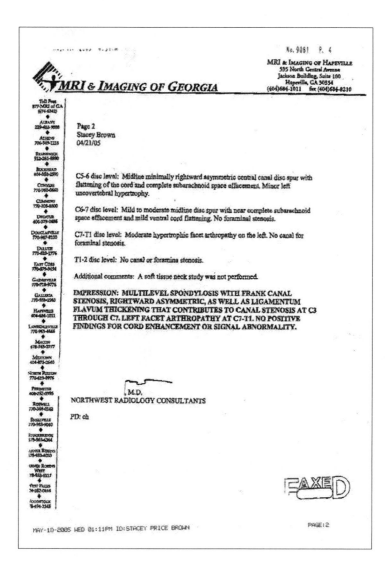

MRI & IMAGING OF GEORGIA

MRI & IMAGING OF HAPEVILLE
595 North Central Avenue
Jackson Building, Suite 100
Hapeville, GA 30354
(404)684-1011   fax (404)684-8210

Toll Free
877-MRI of GA
(674-6342)

ALBANY
229-431-9558

ATHENS
706-549-1223

BRUNSWICK
912-261-8890

BUCKHEAD
404-350-2890

CONYERS
770-760-0660

CUMMING
770-205-8800

DECATUR
404-379-0886

DOUGLASVILLE
770-947-8100

DULUTH
770-623-1776

EAST COBB
770-579-0434

GAINESVILLE
770-718-9775

GALLERIA
770-859-1963

HAPEVILLE
404-684-1011

LAWRENCEVILLE
770-963-4465

MACON
478-745-2777

MIDTOWN
404-872-0640

NORTH FULTON
770-623-8975

PREMIERE
404-252-0595

ROSWELL
770-368-0242

SNELLVILLE
770-985-9060

STOCKBRIDGE
175-865-4264

WARNER ROBINS
478-953-8213

WARNER ROBINS
WEST
78-953-8117

WEST PACES
34-352-0644

WOODSTOCK
8-694-3343

Page 2
Stacey Brown
04/21/05

C5-6 disc level: Midline minimally rightward asymmetric central canal disc spur with
flattening of the cord and complete subarachnoid space effacement. Minor left
uncovertebral hypertrophy.

C6-7 disc level: Mild to moderate midline disc spur with near complete subarachnoid
space effacement and mild ventral cord flattening. No foraminal stenosis.

C7-T1 disc level: Moderate hypertrophic facet arthropathy on the left. No canal for
foraminal stenosis.

T1-2 disc level: No canal or foramina stenosis.

Additional comments: A soft tissue neck study was not performed.

IMPRESSION: MULTILEVEL SPONDYLOSIS WITH FRANK CANAL
STENOSIS, RIGHTWARD ASYMMETRIC, AS WELL AS LIGAMENTUM
FLAVUM THICKENING THAT CONTRIBUTES TO CANAL STENOSIS AT C3
THROUGH C7. LEFT FACET ARTHROPATHY AT C7-T1. NO POSITIVE
FINDINGS FOR CORD ENHANCEMENT OR SIGNAL ABNORMALITY.

M.D.
NORTHWEST RADIOLOGY CONSULTANTS

PD: ch

FAXED

The MRI of Lumbar Spine Taken August 8, 2006

The lumbar spine shows degenerative bulging and anular tears, with
no high signal. When there is no high signal, this is an indication that
there is disc disruption along the spine. It is called a high-intensity zone
for chronic pain. When I viewed my film, the disc in question showed
complete desiccation, and the disc was completely black.

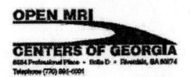

OPEN MRI

CENTERS OF GEORGIA
6684 Professional Place • Suite D • Riverdale, GA 30274
Telephone (770) 991-6901

NAME: **PRICE-BROWN, STACEY**
MEDICAL RECORD#:   **0001257**
DATE OF BIRTH: 05/23/1959
REFERRING DOCTOR: M.D.
EXAM DATE: 08/08/2006
EXAM NAME: **MRI OF THE LUMBAR SPINE**

HISTORY: MS, DEGENERATIVE JOINT DISEASE

TECHNIQUE: Views of the lumbar spine in all three orthogonal planes.

No prior comparisons studies

FINDINGS:

L5-S1: Mild degenerative disc with maintained height, but loss of signal. Midline disco-protrusion seen on both T2 and T1 weighted sagittal images with midline protrusion and small focus of outer annular high signal indicative of tear. Significant neural compressive effect is not present. Normal posterior elements. The foramen are widely patent.

L4-5: Normal.

L3-4: Shows very mild degenerative bulging with no neural compressive effects.

L2-3 and other levels are normal. The conus and cauda equina are unremarkable.

IMPRESSION:

1. L5-S1: Central focal noncompressive protrusion very likely the cause of pain. No high signal, foci or atrophy in the conus to suggest distal changes of MS.

_____
M.D.

CHAPTER SEVENTEEN

Lymphomatoid Papulosis/Cutaneous T Cell Lymphoma

Cancer does not discriminate. It has revealed some of its secrets to our medical professionals, but apparently not enough. It may not allow one to know it's there sometimes until it's too late. I am all too familiar with its impact on my family. My father was a Marlboro man! He was diagnosed with lung cancer, which, by the time it was diagnosed, had metastasized; that is, the tumor causing the lung cancer had moved to the bone. He passed away six weeks after diagnosis.

Sarcomas are unusual types of tumors in that they occur in any site in the human body. A sarcoma is a malignant or cancerous soft tissue tumor that originates in tissue such as fat, muscle, nerves, tendons, and blood and lymph vessels. However, these types of cancerous tumors can also be found in the bone and are called osteosarcomas. As it happened, the tumor started in my father's lung and metastasized to his shoulder, so he had both types of sarcomas: soft tissue and osteo. God was merciful, and he ultimately died of a massive stroke. My father suffered, but he didn't suffer long. He refused treatment. His reasoning was this: the doctor had already advised him that the cancer had already metastasized and there was nothing they could do for him, so why bother? He wanted to die with dignity. My father did not believe in drugs, so he didn't take any—no pain killers, not even an aspirin. He refused any and all treatment right up to the end. God bless him!

There are many different types of cancer. There are the common types that we are familiar with, the types that we are warned of receiving if we smoke too much or from secondhand smoke such as lung cancer. The most common form of cancer among women is undetected breast, ovarian, and cervical cancers. This is why we now have extensive campaigns for early detection. Death from these forms of cancer can be prevented. We urge people not to smoke, and we now know that secondhand smoke kills. Early detection with a regular breast examination or a Pap smear saves lives. We urge men to seek prostate exams and colon exams; yet, in spite of all we do to prevent death and in spite of what we know, there are still a number of people who refuse to seek early detection. Unfortunately, there is a deadly form of cancer that still claims the lives of over five thousand children each year, and its name is leukemia. It is a cancer of the blood-forming tissues.

What we know about cancer is that all cancers originate in living cells. All forms of life, plants, animals, and man consists of living cells; and, as such, it stands to reason that cancer can exist in and has been observed in many forms of plant and animal life, as well as in man. As living things grow from inception, the process of cell division is called mitosis. One cell becomes two, two into four, four becomes eight, and the process continues until the number of cells are needed that God ordained to form

The following is an illustration of cutaneous T cell lymphoma and pretty much what my hands and feet looked like.

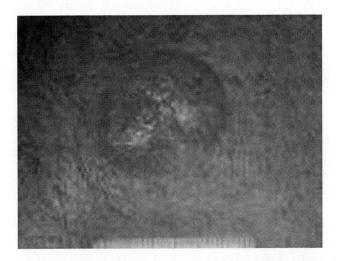

tissue. You get the picture. Normally, mitosis is controlled naturally to replace cells as the body ages or grows or is injured, so that the body produces only the kinds and amounts of cells it needs. The process of mitosis is highly regulated by a process called cell death. When anything interferes with control, the cells grow without stopping. These masses of tissue are called tumors. When the tumors are self-contained, they are called benign tumors and can be removed surgically without growing back or affecting or invading surrounding tissue. If a tumor is malignant, it is one that is not self-contained. That is, it is one that will invade surrounding tissue and set up new growths in parts of the body nowhere near the original site of the tumor. This process is called metastasis, and the new tumors are called metastases.

Cancer is known as the silent killer. There is little or no warning in the early stages. Early detection is the best chance for survival. There are many common forms of cancer; however, there are several forms that are rare and difficult to detect. What if your cancer doctor knew nothing about your rare form of cancer? What if he should have been aware of your textbook condition and still refused to help you even after you asked for an x-ray and there was not even the slightest bit of procedural curiosity? Then this is an outrage. This is still happening.

I was waiting to see my oncologist/hematologist, and a woman sitting next to me struck up a conversation. She advised me that she was terminally ill. I could tell from the matter-of-factness of her statement that she was still not over the shock of the news of her illness, and from the tears immediately welling up in my eyes her bold statement had certainly impacted me. She continued to advise me that she had been seeing her primary care physician repeatedly for what she had been initially diagnosed for what she thought was emphysema. She continued to return to him, advising him that the medication and steroids were not working and that she was getting progressively worse and that she was beginning to cough and bring up blood. She asked him, begged him, to do a simple x-ray, and he refused and told her to continue to take her medication and give it a chance to work. As she continued with her story, telling me that the cough got worse, that's when I noticed the raspy tone to her voice. She finally decided enough was enough and sought a second opinion. She told me that the second doctor took one look at the x-ray in complete disgust and advised her that she had bronchial cancer, which could have been easily detected, treated, and cured if the first doctor had heeded her cries to take an x-ray at the outset. I realized at that moment that my mouth had dropped open, and I had to will myself to close it. She continued to talk, oblivious as to whether I was listening or not; she just needed to vent. I interrupted her and told her she should sue that buffoon for everything he's worth. Her eyes dropped, and there was an uncomfortable silence. She told me with gentleness in her voice that all the money in the world cannot replace her life. I felt so foolish and realized at that moment that her only concern was the quality of time she had left with her children and grandchildren, and that's all that mattered! We are a litigious society and have lost our way.

On June 20, 2002, I woke up with two tender pustules on the palm of my left hand. One was in the center and the other was near the wrist. I immediately went to see my primary care physician. There was nothing to prepare me for what was about to transpire over the next few weeks. He speculated that it might be something called foot-and-mouth disease. I laughed in light of the fact that mad cow disease was making headlines. Maybe the cow had brain cancer. Of course, there was nothing funny about what was happening to me. He advised me that he did not know what was wrong with me and had to refer me to a dermatologist. My primary care physician is an excellent doctor because he knows that he doesn't know and made arrangements for me to be seen by the dermatologist in two days. By the next morning the two increased to around ten and were no longer contained to the left palm. Whatever was happening had now spread to both hands and to the bottom of both my feet. By June 22, the ten had increased to about fifty and had spread to the bottom of both feet, making it very difficult to walk. My feet and hands were swollen, and the pustules had become extremely tender, and some were dry and scaly in places. I was beginning to look as if I was mutating, and my hands and feet could have easily been used in a science fiction production.

Once I had arrived at the dermatologist's office, I was placed under the care of a physician's assistant. She was very kind and very knowledgeable. Although it had only been two days, she noted that the pustules were multiplying and healing rapidly. The healed pustules would leave a scaly brown appearance. Fresh pustules were replacing the healed pustules as quickly as they were healing. She indicated that she would have to take a punch biopsy of fresh pustules in order to confirm her suspicions. She would not tell me what she suspected so as not to alarm me. Initially she took a 3 mm punch biopsy on the plantar surface of my right foot and opted to defer treatment until we knew what we were dealing with. Initially, there were breakouts on the palms of my hands, but she had to follow procedure. The test results came back showing mixed infiltrates including lymphocytes, neutrophils, and atypical lymphocytes. Neutrophils are the first cells to respond when there is an infection or injury. Their targets are bacteria, fungi, protozoa, viruses, virally infected cells, and tumor cells. They develop in bone marrow and take about two weeks to mature. There was also the presence of tinea or athlete's foot on the plantar surface—how embarrassing. I was treated for tinea and then fresh tissue had to be obtained for an immunohistochemistry.

An immunohistochemistry is a test used to detect the presence of specific proteins in cells or tissues, and is widely used for the diagnosis of cancer, since cancers originate within a single cell and they can be classified by the type of cell in which it originates and by the location of the cell. Carcinomas originate in epithelial cells: the skin, digestive tract, glands, etc. Leukemia starts in bone marrow and stem cells or, as previously indicated, blood-forming tissue. Lymphoma originates in lymphatic tissue, whereas melanoma arises in melanocytes. Teratoma is cancer that begins within germ cells. As such, specific markers are used to detect cancer. CD15 and CD30 are the markers used to detect Hodgkin's disease. If the doctor suspected colon cancer, for example, then he would have been looking for a specific antigen called CEA or carcino-embryonic antigen. Atypical lymphocytes are lymphocytes that have become quite large and are easily discernable under a microscope.

Gene-rearrangement studies had to be performed, which could only be done at the University Hospital in order to rule out the possibility of a lymphomatous infiltrate. The gene rearrangement study was a new test developed to determine the presence of lymphoproliferative disease. In other words, they were looking for the presence of cancer, more specifically a rare cancer called cutaneous T cell lymphoma. The medical laboratories at University Hospital were equipped to do the study. In fact, the Emory University is the only hospital in the country equipped to perform this test. Hindsight is always 20/20, but I was blind that weekend. It was all too much to digest. I knew something was terribly wrong by the way my feet and hands looked and the way I felt. It was happening so quickly. The pustules multiplied rapidly. At first there were two and then ten. They turned into twenty and twenty turned into fifty and then one hundred, spreading and healing at lightning speed on both hands and feet. I couldn't believe what was happening. I was back in the dermatologist's office by Monday. The doctor at the laboratory reported that he saw fungi and large atypical lymphs. When these are present, then the presence of a lymphoproliferative disease may also be present. Cancer!

My hands and feet looked like ugly swollen slightly burnt popcorn balls. It was very difficult to walk, and the only exercise I was getting was my husband carrying me outside to the backyard and placing me in our pool. I didn't understand why the pustules were popping up so quickly and then healing and scaling. The physician's assistant was a patient's best friend. Not only was she professional, but also she understood that I was afraid and that I did not understand what was happening to me. She took the time and explained to me as best as she could in layman's terms and then gave me an article to read.

To sum it up, lymphomatoid papulosis or cutaneous T cell lymphoma are characterized by superficial and deep, per vascular and interstitial, mixed-cell infiltrates. Atypical lymphocytes are often present within the epidermis, solitary rather than in nests, and are self-healing. She told me that perhaps the doctors at University Hospital could help me. When the test results were complete, then we would know what we were dealing with. I was referred locally to an oncologist. A total of three-punch biopsies were performed over a period of three months, and the findings were that the doctors at the University Hospital felt the results were inconclusive: not negative and not positive. So what does that mean? Quoting directly from the oncologist's report, the question was posed, "Does this patient have clinical evidence of T cell lymphoma?" By now it was September 30, 2002. Findings from University Hospital showed large atypical cells positive for CD3. The CD3 antigen is highly specific for T cells and is present in majority on mature human T cells, and is a T cell receptor. A neoplasm is any new and abnormal growth of tissue, which is progressive and uncontrolled. I tested positive for the CD30 antigen, which are the primary antibodies used in tandem to differentiate between anaplastic large cell lymphoma and Hodgkin's disease. As you may recall, these are also the markers used in immunohistochemistry. I tested focally positive for CD43 and 45. CD43 is expressed on all thymocytes and T cells. This antibody has been shown useful in identification and classification of T cell malignancies and low-grade B cell lymphomas. CD45 is an antigen present on all human cells, except erythroid cells, platelets, and their precursor cells. CD45 is required for T cell and B cell activation.

A T cell is your body's immune system, your ability to fight disease. Thymocyte cells or T cells are generated in bone marrow. From there, they migrate to the thymus, which is located approximately above your heart for differentiation where the thymus or T cells are further processed. If CD3, CD4, and CD8 T cells do not interact with MHC Class I and II molecules, which bound peptide to the T cells within four days after the T cells mature, then apoptosis will be triggered—cell death. If T cells recognize bound peptides, they further differentiate; otherwise, apoptosis will occur. Further, CD4 and CD8 are co-receptors, and its function is to assist T cells in binding to the correct MHC antigens because there are so many antigen-presenting cells. In plain English, whatever was happening to me was in its early stages. My body was trying to tell me something. I was testing positive. and all the receptors for the disease were present. but nothing was happening so my condition would stand as guarded.

Diagnosis for cutaneous lymphoma in the absence of clinical evidence is difficult. The only evidence presented was the abnormal rash on my hands and feet and the low white count. A gene rearrangement study was ordered in order to differentiate primary cutaneous lymphoma from pseudolymphoma. In light of testing positive for the CD30 antigen and focally positive for CD 43 and 45 I had reason to be concerned. The tests were negative for CD20, which is B cell non-Hodgkin's lymphoma, lysozyme, which protects us from bacterial infection and ALK-1 anaplastic lymphoma kinase, or malignant tumors of the bladder.

The gene rearrangement studies for the T cell receptor gamma gene were inconclusive. So exactly what is a gene rearrangement study? Scientists have learned to take DNA and transpose or rearrange in somatic or body cells. In my case, an immunoglobulin gene rearrangement was conducted; that is, a rearrangement of my body's immune system. The human body contains what are known as 500,000 line one, or L1, elements and out of that amount only eighty can move. There is also another gene rearrangement test called an antibody test where antibodies are assembled by DNA recombination from gene segments in B cells. What this study hopes to prove is how B cells that break the rules of normal gene arrangement may promote autoimmune disease. Again, the results were not negative and not positive, but inconclusive. The doctors at University Hospital felt that the findings were more consistent with a cutaneous CD30-positive T cell lymphoproliferative disorder, which includes a spectrum of disease entities ranging from lymphomatoid papulosis to anaplastic large cell lymphoma. Clinical correlation was recommended for definitive diagnosis—as such, inconclusive. On the medial arch skin biopsy of the left foot, there were large atypical lymphoid cells present, which were termed worrisome, but not diagnostic. Interestingly enough, although the findings were inconclusive, "this does not exclude the possibility of a clonal population." This statement naturally has me concerned. As such it was recommended, in spite of my abnormalities, since I did not clinically demonstrate disseminated lymphoma that I simply follow up in three months and that my condition be left at guarded as of March 3, 2003; but I certainly was not out of the woods.

EMORY MEDICAL LABORATORIES

at Emory University Hospital
1364 Clifton Rd.NE, Atlanta, GA 30322
Phone: 404-712-LABS   Fax: 404-712-0026

EML

Patient: BROWN, STACEY F	**Accession Number:** OH-02-24239
Patient Number:	20

SURGICAL PATHOLOGY CONSULTATION REPORT

SPECIMEN:
  PART 1: RIGHT FOOT

CLINICAL HISTORY:
  43 year old female with a pustular break out on feet and hands. Rule out
  lymphoproliferative disease.

MATERIAL RECEIVED:

  DERMATOPATHOLOGY

  (1) D02-24597 SLIDE/REPORT
  (1) D02-24597 BLOCK
  (1) D02-21879 SLIDE/REPORT &
  (1) D02-24879 BLOCK

MICROSCOPIC DESCRIPTION:
  OSC#D02-21879: The specimen consists of a punch biopsy with epidermis and
  dermis. The epidermis shows mild to moderate acanthosis, focal parakeratosis,
  compact hyperorthokeratosis, and mild intercellular edema associated with
  exocytosis of small lymphocytes. Occasional elongated structures suggestive
  of fungal hyphae are noted in the stratum corneum. The superficial papillary
  dermis shows mild edema and congested thin-walled blood vessels. There is a
  perivascular and interstitial, superficial and deep, mixed inflammatory
  infiltrate of small lymphocytes and large atypical cells admixed with
  scattered histiocytes and neutrophils. Focal red cell extravasation is
  noted. A PAS stain was performed at the outside institution and was reported
  as being positive for fungal hyphae (slide not available for review). Special
  immunohistochemical stains are performed on formalin-fixed, paraffin-embedded
  section. The large atypical cells are positive for CD3, CD30, focally
  positive for CD43 and CD45, but are negative for CD20, lysozyme and ALK-1.

  OSC#D02-24597-A: The specimen consists of a small punch biopsy with epidermis,
  dermis and superficial panniculus. The epidermis shows a thickened compact
  stratum corneum, basal layer pigmentation, focal mild parakeratosis, minimal
  interstitial edema and occasional small lymphocytes along the basal layer. The
  papillary dermis show focal red cell extravasation. A mild superficial
  perivascular inflammatory infiltrate of small lymphocytes and histiocytes is
  present. Scattered large atypical lymphoid cells similar to those seen in the

---

Physician's Copy

CHAPTER EIGHTEEN

Prostaglandins and Platelet Count

It was early spring 2006, and my white count began to slide from mid 3 to low 2. As a result of having leukopenia, my doctor was not too concerned; but as a precaution, a bone marrow biopsy was ordered. Your bone marrow is where your blood cells are created. The blood is the key to life and is the life stream of the human body. The blood produces plasma, red blood cells, white blood cells, and platelets. Plasma makes up 50 percent of the volume of the blood, and is a watery straw-colored liquid. The other parts of the blood float in the plasma. There are many different chemicals, proteins, minerals, and sugars that float around in the plasma; and the chief proteins are called albumin, globulin, and fibrinogen. Red blood cells get their color from hemoglobin, and their function is to carry oxygen and carbon dioxide through the body. As such, red blood cells are constantly moving. White blood cells defend against infection and disease, and are called leukocytes. There are three main types of white blood cells: granulocytes, which constitute the majority of white blood cells at approximately 70 percent; lymphocytes at a rate of 20 percent; and monocytes at a rate of 10 percent. The granulocytes devour bacteria in the blood, and enter infected tissue, and repeat the process. However, if the percentage is deficient, then disease will result. Without granulocytes, infection in the bloodstream will result. This is called blood poisoning or septicemia. Lymphocytes are produced in the lymph glands, and they help the body produce antibodies in order to fight foreign substances or antigens. This is called the body's immunity: the first prostaglandin receptor or GPCR. Monocytes form in the bone marrow and in the spleen, and their function is the same as granulocytes. Platelets repair blood vessels so that the blood doesn't leak out. You always wanted to know what happened when you got a paper cut or when you fell off your bike and Mom was looking for a Band-Aid. The platelets start the clotting process and help repair small blood vessels. In the average human, there are about 200,000 platelets per cubic millimeter of blood. The blood will unlock all the clues to your health. In my case, there were too many variables and not enough answers that made sense, so a bone marrow procedure was ordered by my oncologist.

As you grow, blood cells are produced in the bone marrow and placed in reserve as immature stem cells until they are needed. They are stored in the vertebrae, pelvis, shoulder blades, and ribs. As they mature, they are referred to as blast cells: white blood cells, red blood cells and platelets. White blood cells are part of your immune system and are referred to as leukocytes. Red blood cells are the most abundant in the body, and a lack of these will lead to anemia.

There are five types of white blood cells: lymphocytes, basophils, eosinophils, neutrophils, and monocytes. Eosinophils, neutrophils, and monocytes are called granulocytes. Their job is to destroy bacteria in the body.

Platelets are fragments of the bone marrow megakaryocyte cell, and they contain chemicals that form clots to control bleeding and stimulate the repair of damaged blood vessels. The lack of a sufficient amount of platelets will lead to bruising and bleeding.

When a bone marrow procedure is performed, a doctor will choose to aspirate the tissue from a large bone in order to locate bone marrow for examination. Bone marrow is composed of the spongy tissue found inside the larger bones, and is composed of a fluid and solid portion. There are various bone marrow sites such as the breastbone, hips, spine, and skull, which contain stem cells. Stem cells turn into red and white blood cells and platelets. These are not the same as embryonic stem cells. This procedure offered detailed information about my health. A bone marrow biopsy was performed on an outpatient basis under conscious sedation. In other words, it hurt! In order for them to aspirate the bone marrow for examination, the procedure was extremely painful, and no amount of sedation could have prepared me for a needle being shoved into my hip bone and extracting bone and spongelike material. Conversely, if the procedure were to save my life as a result of early detection, then I would do it again. The results were these: granulocytes 41.8 percent as opposed to a normal 70 percent; monocytes 3.5 percent as opposed to a normal 20 percent; and the only normal reading were the lymphocytes, which read 54.7 percent—higher than the normal rate of 20 percent. My platelets were 355,000 than a normal 200,000, so what my body was revealing was an imbalance.

In a study conducted by the HEJ Research Institute of Chemistry on the therapeutic use of inhibitors and anti-inflammatory drugs, its findings were that the effects of chemistry, metabolism, and pharmacology and its effects on **prostaglandins,** prostacylcins, Thromboxane A2, and leukatrines cause leukematic blast cells to accumulate in the bone marrow and suppress the growth and differentiation of normal haemopoietic cells. Leukemic cells proliferate primarily in the bone marrow and lymphoid tissue where they interfere with normal haemopoesis and immunity. Red blood cells or erythrocytes transport oxygen in the blood. As red blood cells form in the bone marrow, it loses the nucleus. This process is called **haemopoesis.** During this process, it carries more hemoglobin because of the loss of the nucleus. From there, they migrate from the bone marrow to the blood and infiltrate healthy tissue.

A pathologist can make a determination by looking for abnormal cells in the blood. These cells tell a story, and, without proper training and experience, they would not know what they were looking for. Myelodysplasia is a rare disease with only 15 to 20,000 new cases being diagnosed each year in the United States. It has been given the name MDS, or myelodysplasiac syndrome. **Myelodysplasia** refers to a group of disorders in which the bone marrow does not function normally and produces an insufficient number of cells. This disease generally affects males more than females, and the median age is 60; but it also affects children, usually less than one hundred a year. The disease usually progresses into acute myeloid leukemia. The disease begins with the presence of anemia, neutropenia, and a reduced number of white cells circulating in the bloodstream; and it eventually affects the person's ability to produce normal cells, hence the low white cell, red cell, and platelet counts. The patient will present with complaints of chest pain and difficulty breathing, chronic fatigue, and complaints of feeling cold or chilled. As the disease progresses, abnormal granules will present in the cells. Almost half of patient death is the result of infection or prolonged bleeding after the disease progresses to acute myelogenous leukemia. A low platelet count increases the susceptibility to bleeding, and this condition is called **thrombocytopenia**. In my case, my test results are constant for a high platelet count. This condition is called **thrombocytosis**. A high platelet count can occur for several reasons. The presence of an inflammatory disease or autoimmune disease in the body (I have several) after surgery or after an accident will increase the platelet count as a defense mechanism. Some cancers will cause a high platelet count, such as bowel cancer; however, a high platelet count can be seen in patients with myelodysplasiac syndrome. In certain subtypes of this disease, there will be a high platelet count; and again, it takes a trained physician to know the difference in order to save the patient's life, because this subtype is rare.

The jury is still out as to whether or not this blood disorder is a form of cancer. In 1990, the World Health Organization put this disease into eight subtypes because it is so difficult to classify. The classifications were based upon the patient having refractory anemia, the presence of circulating white cells, low iron levels and platelet levels. The combinations of these factors were put into a formula to determine an outcome: early emerging myelodysplasia.

In order to understand the disease, we must first understand how cells are formed. While you are in your mother's womb, blood cells are being formed primarily in your liver and spleen, and other cells develop in the thymus, lymph nodes, and bone marrow. This process is called **hemopoeisis**. These are the **embryonic stem cells** that scientists are seeking for genetic purposes. They are called the formed elements or the growth factors of the human body. After birth, the process is limited to the bone marrow, and some of the white blood cells are produced in lymphoid tissue. A **blast** is an immature blood cell, which forms in the bone marrow. A **fibroblast** is a cell responding to increased growth factors from abnormal megakaryocytes. **Megakaryocytes** are large bone marrow cells with a lobulate (lobe-shaped) nucleus that is the precursor to blood platelets. In other words, fibroblasts are cells that respond to connective tissue. Connective tissue includes fibrous, reticular, cartilage, and bone tissue, the vascular matrix of the body, adipose tissue (fat), and the supporting and connecting structures of the body. Usually diagnosis involves laboratory evidence of circulating immature myeloid and erythroid cells. All types of cells develop from a "master cell" in the body, which can tell a story as to the condition of the health of the individual. These cells generate other differentiated cell types. Each tissue in the body contains a unique type of stem cell that renews and replaces that tissue. As a result of wear and tear, damage or disease, these cells generate other cells in the body. As such, new cells will replace other cells as a result of wear or tear, and abnormal cells will appear as a result of disease.

There are seven different cell lines, each controlled by a specific growth factor. A growth factor is the substance that promotes the growth of cells. For example, when you are cut there is an epidermal growth factor, which is known as EGF. If there is an abnormality, as previously discussed, then there will be a fibroblast growth factor known as FGF and normal cell growth known as hematopoietic cell growth factor, or HCGF. Then it stands to reason that a tumor, for example, will produce large amounts of growth factors. From the seven different cell lines, a cell divides, producing a daughter. The daughter remains a stem cell, and the other becomes a precursor cell: lymphoid or myeloid. Lymphoid pertains to the lymphatic system; however, myeloid pertains to the bone marrow and the **spinal cord**. (Remember the receptor of prostaglandins acting on the spinal cord.) These cells will continue to develop into mature blood cells, or leukemia may develop at any point in cell differentiation.

As aforementioned, diagnosis of an abnormality begins with finding evidence of circulating immature myeloid and erythroid cells. As indicated in my report, the findings were positive for myeloid cells to erythroid cells at a ratio of 3 to1. Leukemic cells accumulate in the bone marrow and replace normal blood cells and spread to the liver, spleen, lymph nodes, central nervous system, gonads, and kidneys, earning the name *myeloid* because it destroys the cells in the bone marrow. As such, the disease, myelodysplasia, can eventually turn into acute myeloid leukemia. A chronic myeloproliferative disorder is characterized by a myeloid cell lineage. The erythroid cells are progenitor cell lines for leukemia. The next level of diagnosis is that there will be a slight increase in bone marrow reticulin fibers without any known cause. My report notes a slight increase in reticulin fibers. Myelodysplasia is also known as the pre-leukemia. The other conditions associated with this disease are ineffective production of blood cells. My diagnostic report noted that my B cells are sparse. Other associated abnormalities are neutropenia, leukopenia, anemia, and thrombocytopenia. Based upon the diagnostic evidence, there was a finding that "early emerging myelodysplasia cannot be ruled out based on the available material." However, it should be noted that myelodysplasia can also be diagnosed as the result of an individual having preexisting rare genetic disorders.

This is an illustration of the lymphatic system. These are the tissues and organs that produce, carry, and store white blood cells in the human body.

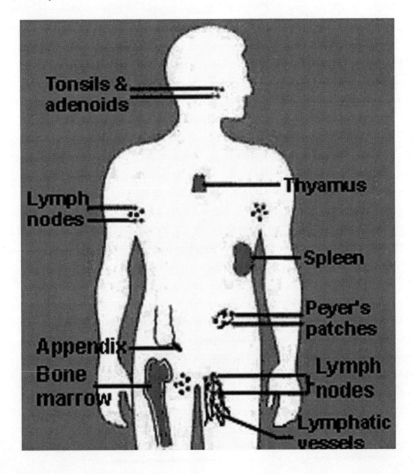

RTE: USIAPS SEQ: ACCR

DIANON SYSTEMS

HEMATOPATHOLOGY REPORT

Connecticut Lic. #: CL-0356

Accession No.	Chart No.	Sex	D.O.B.	Page
SA0003		F	05/23/1959 46 Yrs	1 of 2

Patient Name	Collected
PRICE, STACEY P	03/16/06

Requesting Physician	Received
	03/17/06

	Reported
	03/21/06

Indications For Study

ASCCR01   DIAGNOSTIC REPORT

CANCER CARE
TH

FINAL DIAGNOSIS

PHOTOMICROGRAPH

1 - BIOPSY, NORMOCELLULAR MARROW
2 - BIOPSY, TRILINEAGE HEMATOPOIESIS

Peripheral Blood
(CBC DATA ONLY):

1. Mild leukopenia/neutropenia.

Bone Marrow
1. Essentially normocellular marrow for age with maturing trilineage hematopoiesis, see comment.

myelodysplasia,

3. Limited iron stain studies, see description below.

4. Focal slight increase in reticulin fibers.

Comment
Recommend exclusion of secondary etiologies for the mild leukopenia/neutropenia seen in this patient. High-grade myelodysplasia is not detected on this biopsy. However, an early/emerging myelodysplasia cannot be ruled out based on the available material. Correlation with additional pertinent clinical and laboratory data such as morphologic examination of freshly prepared bone marrow aspirate smears, cytogenetic analysis results, peripheral blood smear features, etc., and patient follow-up are recommended. Should you have any questions, I can be reached at

Clinical Information
46 year old female with leukopenia, rule out MDS. The provided ICD-9 code indicates lymphoma (202.80).

Gross Description
BONE MARROW CORE:
Received in formalin is a homogeneous bone marrow core measuring 1.3 cm in length x 0.2 cm in diameter. Specimen is submitted in toto in 1 cassette. Associated clot measures 0.7 X 0.3 X 0.2 cm and is submitted in the same cassette. The specimen has been decalcified to reduce fragmentation during sectioning.

CANCER CARE

Price, Stacey P
Patient Account #
Date: 03-03-2006 07:40:00

ID: 35208   03-03-06
CVWB   10:46
                                 Patient
                                 Limits 3
WBC   2.7 L x10^3/uL   4.5   10.5
LY   55.6 H %   20.5   51.1
MO   4.8 M %   1.7   9.3
GR   39.6 ML %   42.2   75.2
LY#   1.5   x10^3/uL   1.2   3.4
MO#   0.1 M x10^3/uL   0.1   0.6
GR#   1.1 ML x10^3/uL   1.4   6.5
RBC   4.53   x10^6/uL   4.00   6.00
Hgb   12.1   g/dL   11.0   18.0
Hct   36.9   %   35.0   60.0
MCV   81.5   fL   80.0   99.9
MCH   26.7 L pg   27.0   31.0
MCHC 32.8 L g/dL   33.0   37.0
RDW   14.5 H %   11.6   13.7
Plt 303.   x10^3/uL   150.   450.
MPV   6.2 L fL   7.8   11.0

WBC HISTOGRAM   RBC HISTOGRAM   PLT HISTOGRAM

CHAPTER NINETEEN

Leukopenia/CBC

In September 2004, I complained of a sore throat. Although my tonsils had been removed, it was difficult to swallow, and my throat was inflamed and covered with mucous. I was coughing up phlegm with blood. My doctor immediately knew something was wrong. Upon examination he noted that the lymph nodes were swollen asymmetrically on the right side of the throat. He immediately knew this was a red flag because of the pattern of swelling. The vessels in my nose were at their limits and had burst, which accounted for the blood in my throat for four days. My primary care physician is a true professional who cares about his patients because he took the time to explain to me why I was coughing up globs of blood. He reassured me that the blood was not coming from my lungs. He explained how the vessels in the nose get infected, swell, burst, and bleed, and that mine were draining at the back of the throat. I was coughing it up instead of at the front of the nose where it would have resulted in a nosebleed. He was just as prudent to refer me to an oncologist because of the asymmetric swelling. I was back in the hands of the oncologist. Upon initial examination, it was determined that nodes were still palpable even after antibiotic treatment; but I was advised that this was common after only two weeks of antibiotic treatment and that a few more weeks should give the medicine enough time to reduce the nodes in the neck and throat. My condition was again listed as guarded, and a four-week return visit was ordered. When I returned for my follow-up visit, the nodes were still palpable asymmetrically on the right side of the throat and, additionally, a lymph node under the left arm was flaring up and was palpable. The reason I knew it was there was that it was painful and palpitating. The blood work revealed a low white blood count and anemia in spite of the medicine taken to prevent this condition, and I was also complaining of abdominal pain. I was referred to an endocrinologist. He ordered a colonoscopy and abdominal scan. Both were negative, thank God. The anemia mystery remains to date even after a hysterectomy. Then on Wednesday, January 19, 2005, I was back in my primary care physician's office because I was bringing up the globs again, and I could feel the swelling in my throat. He again suspected leukopenia or lymphoma. My white count had bottomed out to 2.7, and to this day I am having unresolved leukopenia and anemia.

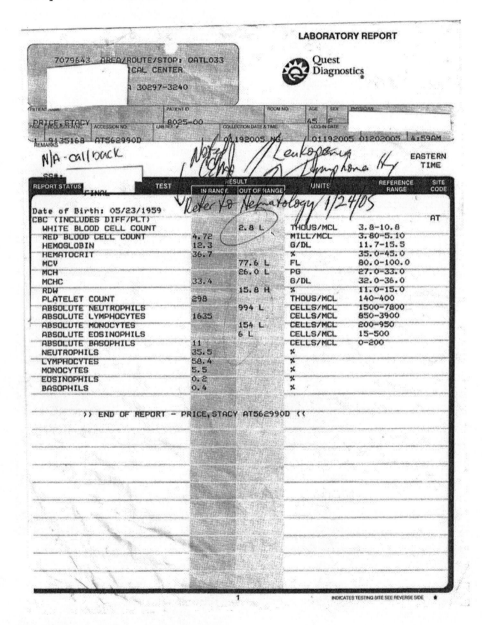

LABORATORY REPORT

7079643 AREA/ROUTE/STOP: OATL033
CAL CENTER
30297-3240

Quest Diagnostics

PRICE, STACY   PATIENT ID 8025-00   AGE 45   SEX F

9135168   ATS62990D   01192005   01192005 01202005 14:59AM

N/A - call back   EASTERN TIME

REPORT STATUS: FINAL

TEST	RESULT IN RANGE	RESULT OUT OF RANGE	UNITS	REFERENCE RANGE	SITE CODE
Date of Birth: 05/23/1959					
CBC (INCLUDES DIFF/PLT)					AT
WHITE BLOOD CELL COUNT		2.8 L	THOUS/MCL	3.8-10.8	
RED BLOOD CELL COUNT	4.72		MILL/MCL	3.80-5.10	
HEMOGLOBIN	12.3		G/DL	11.7-15.5	
HEMATOCRIT	36.7		%	35.0-45.0	
MCV		77.6 L	FL	80.0-100.0	
MCH		26.0 L	PG	27.0-33.0	
MCHC	33.4		G/DL	32.0-36.0	
RDW		15.8 H	%	11.0-15.0	
PLATELET COUNT	298		THOUS/MCL	140-400	
ABSOLUTE NEUTROPHILS		994 L	CELLS/MCL	1500-7800	
ABSOLUTE LYMPHOCYTES	1635		CELLS/MCL	850-3900	
ABSOLUTE MONOCYTES		154 L	CELLS/MCL	200-950	
ABSOLUTE EOSINOPHILS		6 L	CELLS/MCL	15-500	
ABSOLUTE BASOPHILS	11		CELLS/MCL	0-200	
NEUTROPHILS	35.5		%		
LYMPHOCYTES	58.4		%		
MONOCYTES	5.5		%		
EOSINOPHILS	0.2		%		
BASOPHILS	0.4		%		

>> END OF REPORT - PRICE, STACY ATS62990D <<

INDICATES TESTING SITE SEE REVERSE SIDE

1

Leukopenia is an autoimmune disease. Neutropenia, also an autoimmune disease, describes a condition where mature neutrophils, or their precursors, lead to cell destruction and reduced blood neutrophil cell count. Leukopenia occurs when the total white blood cell count is reduced to less than 4,000 cells per deciliter. Cell production occurs in the bone marrow. Leukopenia also suggests the presence of rare disorders. Leukopenia often implies neutropenia and other pathologic conditions where the bone marrow does not produce enough neutrophils, basophils, lymphocytes, and eosinophils. In order to understand this disease, we must first understand what a blood count is.

This condition may be caused by an autoimmune disease or common medications used in an attempt to cure the disease or alleviate the symptoms of the disease. It is a common occurrence in pain management and can be caused by medications such as those used to cure gastrointestinal tract or digestive system disorders, cardiovascular drugs such as beta blockers, drugs affecting blood pressure, anticoagulants, diuretics, drugs affecting the central nervous system such as those used with multiple sclerosis, antihistamines, antidepressants, NSAIDS, COX-2 inhibitors, muscle relaxers, opiates etc.

A complete blood count, or CBC for short, will test for every component in the blood including the platelet count, white blood cells, and red blood cells. White blood cell counts vary slightly from laboratory to laboratory but are generally between 4,300 to 10,800 cells per liter or 4.3 to 10.8 as a normal measure. There are different types of white blood cells in your body, and a machine called an automated white cell differential will split the white cells up into their categories using percentages or differentials. There are six white cell categories: granulocytes, lymphocytes, monocytes, eosinophils, neutrophils, and basophils. In order to be diagnosed with leukopenia, there is a deficiency in at least one of the aforementioned categories. Each one of the six white cell categories plays a unique role in the immune system. Granulocytes or mast cells are fixed in tissues and initiate the inflammatory response. Lymphocytes produce antibodies and regulate immune responses. Monocytes are like little soldiers. They capture infecting organisms for identification, ingest them, and remove damaged or dying cells and cell debris. When monocytes become fixed in tissue, they are called macrophages. It is the duty of the eosinophils to kill infecting parasites and produce allergic reactions. If you will note in my sample report, my absolute eosinophils count reported was 0.2. Neutrophils identify and kill infecting organisms and remove dead tissue. Basophils circulate in the blood and initiate the inflammatory response. In this particular report dated March 15, 2005, my overall white blood count was 3.5. However, in the report dated February 28, 2005, my overall white blood count was 2.5.

QUEST DIAGNOSTICS INCORPORATED
CLIENT SERVICE

SPECIMEN INFORMATION
SPECIMEN: AT456180E
REQUISITION: 1647547

COLLECTED: 02/28/2005
RECEIVED: 02/28/2005   21:41 ET
REPORTED: 03/01/2005   05:19 ET

PATIENT INFORMATION
BROWN,STACY

DOB: 05/23/1959 AGE: 45
GENDER: F
SSN:
ID: 10/579
PHONE:

REPORT STATUS FINAL

ORDERING PHYSICIAN

CLIENT INFORMATION
A75418   ^QTL832

                          _DOR

Test Name	In Range	Out of Range		Reference Range	Lab
HEPATIC FUNCTION PANEL					AT
PROTEIN, TOTAL	7.4			6.0-8.3 G/DL	
ALBUMIN	4.5			3.5-4.9 G/DL	
GLOBULIN	2.9			2.2-4.2 G/DL (CALC)	
ALBUMIN/GLOBULIN RATIO	1.6			0.8-2.0 (CALC)	
BILIRUBIN, TOTAL	0.3			0.2-1.3 MG/DL	
BILIRUBIN, DIRECT	0.1			0.0-0.3 MG/DL	
BILIRUBIN, INDIRECT	0.2			0.0-1.3 MG/DL (CALC)	
ALKALINE PHOSPHATASE	71			20-125 U/L	
AST	18			2-35 U/L	
ALT	15			2-40 U/L	
HEMOGRAM/PLT					AT
WHITE BLOOD CELL COUNT		2.5	L	3.8-10.8 THOUS/MCL	
RED BLOOD CELL COUNT	5.02			3.80-5.10 MILL/MCL	
HEMOGLOBIN	12.8			11.7-15.5 G/DL	
HEMATOCRIT	40.0			35.0-45.0 %	
MCV		79.6	L	80.0-100.0 FL	
MCH		25.5	L	27.0-33.0 PG	
MCHC	32.0			32.0-36.0 G/DL	
RDW		17.0	H	11.0-15.0 %	
PLATELET COUNT	260			140-400 THOUS/MCL	

PERFORMING LABORATORY INFORMATION
AT   QUEST DIAGNOSTICS-ATLANTA,   E. TUCKER, GA 30084
     Laboratory Director: YYY   M

BROWN,STACY - AT456180E   Page 1 - End of Report

Complete Blood Count/Anemia

Have you ever had a blood test, received a report, and wondered what all the letters stand for? The red blood count measures the number of red blood cells in the blood, and the normal range is 4.2 to 5.9 million cells. This number will vary slightly from each laboratory. The hemoglobin measures the amount of protein found in the blood. Hemoglobin is what carries oxygen in the blood, and the normal range is 13 to 18 grams per deciliter for men and 12 to 16 for women. Hematocrit measures the ratio of the volume of red blood cells to the volume of whole blood. The normal range for women is 37 to 48 percent, and for men is 45 to 52 percent. MCV stands for mean cell volume. That is the average volume of a red cell. For example, the normal range is 86-98 femtoliters. My MCV averaged 77.6, which is low. This indicates to the person reading the reports that not only are my red blood cells low in number, but I am also anemic. MCH stands for mean cell hemoglobin. It indicates the amount of hemoglobin in the average red cell. MCHC stands for mean cell hemoglobin concentration in the average concentration of hemoglobin in a given volume of red cells. The normal range is 32 to 36 percent. RDW stands for red cell distribution width, and measures the variability of the size of red blood cells. The normal range is between 11 and 15. Platelet count measures the number of platelets in a volume of blood, and plays a vital role in blood clotting. This information is vital if you are about to have surgery. The normal range for a platelet count is 150,000 to 400,000.

If there is a deficiency of red blood cells, then this condition is called anemia. Anemia will occur for any of three reasons: blood loss, destruction of red blood cells, or inadequate production from bone marrow. In some cases, in may be genetic such as sickle cell, or it may be caused by medication. This condition is called autoimmune hemolytic anemia, whereby antibiotics or antiseizure medication causes the body to mistake red blood cells for foreign invaders. Aplastic anemia occurs when the bone marrow is unable to produce sufficient numbers of blood cells. This is caused by medication and viral infections. Chronic diseases of other organs can also cause aplastic anemia because the bone marrow is needed to produce red blood cells to fight infection and disease.

CHAPTER TWENTY

Neutropenia

Neutrophils were placed in the blood to fight bacteria. It is a type of white blood cell. When doctors make a diagnosis of neutropenia, then they are describing a state rather than a condition. Allow me to explain. It is an autoimmune disease, and it describes an underlying condition whereby there is an abnormally low number of neutrophils found in the blood, and this condition remains constant. It indicates that there is the risk of severe infection in the blood, kidneys, lungs, mouth, throat, sinuses, ears, and skin because the bone marrow is not producing enough neutrophils. The lower the neutrophil count, the greater the risk of infection. This condition is more common in women than in men. Cancer patients with neutropenia are considered among the high-risk groups for complications and mortality associated with this disease. Periodontal disease, fungal or bacterial pneumonia also may be a result of this disease. Although this is a rare condition, it is common in African Americans and Yemenite Jews. Neutropenia is caused by the destruction of neutrophils after they are produced as a result of drug toxicity, vitamin deficiency, blood diseases, virus diseases, and bone marrow disorders. Neutropenia can also occur, for example, after heart surgery, because white blood cells will pool causing infection. A determination of neutropenia will occur when a neutrophil count is below 2,000. The average white blood count for a healthy individual is 3,650 for neutrophils, 2,500 lymphocytes, 430 monocytes, 150 eosinophils, and 30 basophils.

CHAPTER TWENTY-ONE

Migraine Headaches

Many people suffer from migraine headaches, and some have suffered for years before they sought professional help. They are extremely debilitating and can rob you of days of function at a time. The brain is still a mystery, and scientists still don't know what causes migraines; but they postulate that when the trigeminal nerve that runs through the brain is stimulated, then serotonin levels drop, resulting in a migraine headache. The trigeminal nerve is a major pain pathway in your nerve system. Serotonin is an organic compound that can be found in the bloodstream and human tissue, and it is capable of raising blood pressure. A headache can be triggered by smell, light, loud noise, stress, or lack of rest. When a headache is taking place, then serotonin levels drop, and this causes the trigeminal nerve to release neuropeptides, which travel to your brain's outer covering. This is why it feels as if your head is about to explode. Neuropeptides are any variety of peptides found in neural tissue. A peptide is a molecule, and a molecule has chemical properties. Basically, neuropeptides release chemical properties into brain tissue, resulting in a headache.

Once neuropeptides reach the brain's outer covering, they cause the blood vessels to become dilated and inflamed, resulting in headache pain. Remember at the beginning of the book I discussed peptides in the stomach. There is a correlation between the stomach, hunger, and headache pain.

It has been determined that there are more women migraine sufferers than men. Studies have revealed imbalances in levels of magnesium have caused nerve cells in the brain to misfire, resulting in headache pain. Women have a higher level of estrogen and progesterone, and fluctuations immediately before and during the onset of menstruation have been reported. My experience has been that food worsens migraines, and studies have shown that alcohol, beer, red wine, aged cheeses, chocolate, fermented, pickled, or marinated food, MSG, or even waiting too long to eat can bring on a migraine headache.

The difference between a migraine headache and a regular headache is that a migraine is concentrated on one side of the head and is often accompanied by nausea, vomiting, and blurred vision; and it is a headache that recurs. A migraine involves major neurological involvement and may be mistaken for a stroke or symptoms of multiple sclerosis such as speech difficulty, confusion, and weakness in an arm or leg, and tingling of the face and hands, or temporary loss of vision. During an attack, you may experience increased urination, abdominal pain, mood changes, fatigue, nausea, and vomiting. A simple headache is a hammering, pulsing type of headache that is the result of stress, fever, or high blood pressure. A key element to the cause of migraines is blood flow to the brain. When the arteries constrict, blood flow is reduced, resulting in the pain of a migraine. The way to manage a migraine is to reduce stress, avoid certain foods, and increase rest; but these are just two contributing factors.

There are many migraine medications on the market: over the counter and prescribed. It is a matter of trial and error before you find a fit for your particular situation. I can recall a particular incident where the patient counseling on the pharmacy label simply read, "Use caution when driving or operating machinery, may cause drowsiness, do not mix with alcohol, chew or crush." We see these pharmacy caution labels and read them all of time and take it for granted that the "use caution when operating machinery" is there for drinkers, and I don't drink, so why worry, right? Wrong! The medication is non-narcotic, so what's the big deal, right? Wrong! I was not prepared for this particular side effect when I took over driving on our way back from Orlando, Florida. The drug failed to warn about night vision and peripheral vision. I had just started taking this medication and was not accustomed to it. On our way back to Georgia, the vision in my right eye failed completely. I assumed that "use caution when driving" meant that if the drug made me drowsy, then proper rest and a sufficient amount of coffee would cure that side effect. You know the old saying, "Assumption made an "a**" out of me that night. Thank God my husband didn't go to sleep. He said, "Stacey, can't you see the driver behind you flashing his high beams?" I said, "No." So I signaled and moved out of the fast lane, continued to drive, and a few minutes later his voice remained calm. He said, "Stacey, you're a little close to that guard rail, why don't we stop for coffee?" He had never criticized my driving in the past, so I didn't take it personally; and it was at that moment I realized there was something terribly wrong with my vision. I quickly exited, and it was not until I entered the gas station that I realized my vision was compromised in my right eye. The change had come on slowly while I had been driving and without warning. It was nighttime so the change was not apparent while I had been driving. The only way I can explain what happened is to say that my vision did not blur, but it shadowed over my right eye. If my husband had not observed that something was wrong, the outcome would have been completely different. Needless to say, he drove the rest of the way home. When we returned to Georgia, I went to see an eye doctor, who explained that increased ocular pressure resulting in blurred vision and decreased night vision was a common side effect with this medication. I was sent for an MRI as a precaution to make sure nothing else was wrong, and the scans were normal.

Migraine Headache Sufferer

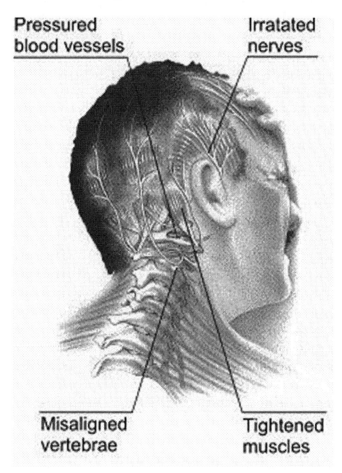

CHAPTER TWENTY-TWO

Lumpectomy: Right Breast/Fibrocystic Breast Disease

It is important for every woman to give herself a breast exam, but sometimes lumps are discovered by happenstance. While performing his own examination, my husband discovered a lump in my right breast, and I immediately had it checked out. I was scheduled for surgery November 12, 2002.

Although a great number of postsurgical biopsies are not cancerous, the fact that I was having surgery and the possibility that it could be cancerous was enough to concern me. As a women's body develops throughout her lifetime, the body undergoes a series of changes from puberty through menopause. Most of the changes in the breast will occur as the body is going through menses or more commonly referred to as your period. Lumps will form in your breast, and an average of 80 percent of these lumps will be benign, which means they are not cancerous, and the rest will be malignant or cancerous. Unfortunately, almost 60 percent of all women have fibrocystic breasts. It is a disease that causes the breasts to be lumpy, painful, and swell, and sometimes discharge fluid from the nipples. If a suspicious lump is discovered, then the doctor will order a lumpectomy. A **lumpectomy** is the removal of a breast lump. It is also referred to as a biopsy. The lump may be either a cyst or breast tissue that has become a solid mass. Fortunately, almost two-thirds of all breast lumps are benign. The chance of malignancy increases with age. When a lump is discovered and removed around or after the time a woman has reached menopause, because of the decrease in the production of hormones, there is an increase in the chance that the lump will be malignant. The surgical procedure is performed when a small incision is made over the lump, and it is removed in one piece. It is then immediately sent to the laboratory for examination. If the lump is benign, then there will be no complications. A malignant tumor requires that you immediately seek the proper follow-up treatment. Any delay may cost you your life. Your must put your faith in God to see you through your trials and then proceed with the procedures.

However, the most important element in your recovery is you. Attitude is everything. It could mean the difference between life and death.

There are different types of tumors, which are distinguishable by their characteristics. Fibroadenomas are solid lumps of fibrous and glandular tissue. It is a benign, moveable tumor and can be felt within the breast tissue. These tumors usually affect women between the ages of eighteen to thirty-five. Papillomas cause a clear or bloody discharge from the nipple. They are wartlike lumps that grow in the lining of the mammary ducts. Breast cancer will announce itself, but not always, with nipple secretions and changes in the appearance of the nipple, as well as dimpling and puckering of the skin. There will be single hard lumps and thickenings, and most often it is painless. Disseminated breast cancer is cancer that has spread undetected to the bones, liver, lungs, and even to the brain. Once the cancer leaves your breast, it is called metastasis, then your survival rate drops by 73 percent. That is why it is *so* important to have regular screenings.

For weeks my left breast began what soon would become a familiar palpitating, annoying, continuous, pulsating alarm to let me know that something was now present.

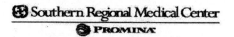

Southern Regional Medical Center
PROMINA

Mammography Department
Riverdale. GA 30274

Date: October 29, 2002   Exam Date: 10/29/2002
                                        ID:

STACEY P. BROWN   Report Sent To:

                    97

Dear Ms. BROWN,

Your mammogram shows an abnormality that requires further evaluation.   We have
sent the mammogram results to the physician, shown above, that you identified on
the day of your appointment. Please contact your physician immediately.

Remember, most abnormalities requiring further evaluation will be one of the many
benign changes that develop in the breast and not cancer.

Your mammogram will become part of your medical file here at Southern Regional
Medical Center for at least 10 years. You are responsible for informing any new
health care provider or mammography facility of the date and location of this
examination.

Sincerely,

                    D.

Radiologist

SURGERY CENTER DISCHARGE INSTRUCTIONS

In order to continue your care at home please follow the instructions checked below.

Date: 11/13/02

1. GENERAL ANESTHESIA OR SEDATION
- Do not drive or operate machinery for 24 hours.
- Do not consume alcohol, tranquilizers, sleeping medications, or any non-prescribed medications for 24 hours.
- Do not make important decisions or sign any important papers in the next 24 hours.
- You should have someone with you tonight at home.
- Children may appear flushed for several hours after surgery.

2. ACTIVITY
- ✓ You are advised to go directly home from the hospital. Restrict your activities and rest for a day. Resume light to normal activity tomorrow. *Right arm*
- You may resume normal activity today. (Do not engage in strenuous activity that may place stress on your incision.)
- Specify activity instructions: _____

3. FLUIDS AND DIET
- Begin with clear liquids, bouillon, dry toast, soda crackers. If not nauseated, you may go to your previous diet when you desire.
- Greasy and spicy foods are not advised.
- ✓ Special diet instructions: *as tolerated*

4. MEDICATIONS
- Prescription sent with you. Use as directed. When taking pain medications, you may experience dizziness or drowsiness. Do not drink alcohol or drive when you are taking these medications.
- You may take a non-prescription "headache remedy" type medication that you normally use, if your surgeon permits, preferably one that does not contain aspirin.
- ✓ You may resume your daily prescription medication schedule.
- Eye kit sent with you.
- ✓ Prescriptions given: _____ , _____ *for pain*

5. OPERATIVE SITE
- ✓ Keep dressing clean and dry. *wear bra for support*
- Do not change dressing.
- ✓ May remove dressing *in 2 days. Leave steri-strips under dressing in place*
- May wash over incision in shower.
- Special instructions: *Bath only. Do not get incision wet*

6. FOLLOW-UP CARE
- ✓ Call your surgeon's office to make an appointment for your post-op check-up. He wants to see you: *1 week*

Call your surgeon if you have any problems that concern you. After office hours, you can reach your physician through his answering service. IF YOU NEED IMMEDIATE ATTENTION COME TO SOUTHERN REGIONAL MEDICAL CENTER'S EMERGENCY DEPT. OR GO TO ANOTHER HOSPITAL NEAR YOUR HOME. Surgery Center's Number is 991-8114 (8:30am - 6:30pm Monday through Friday) if we can answer any questions for you.

CALL YOUR SURGEON FOR ANY OF THE FOLLOWING:
- * Fever over 101 F by mouth.
- * Pain not relieved by medication ordered.
- * Swelling around operative area.
- * Increased redness, warmth, hardness, around operative area.
- * Numb tingling or cold fingers or toes.
- * Blood-soaked dressing (small amounts of oozing may be normal).
- * Increasing and progressive drainage from surgical areas or exam site.
- * If you have not urinated within 6 hours after your surgery, please call your surgeon.

A follow-up call will be attempted by a Surgery Center Nurse to check on your progress. If you have any questions, call your doctor.

COMMENTS: _____

X _____   _____ RN
Patient/Guardian Signature   Nurse Signature
(Rev. 6/2000)

To the contrary, a cancerous growth is **not** tender when touched. When the pain moved to the right side, I knew it was time to get help. On December 6, 2004, another lump was detected in the left breast, and perhaps the pain was sympathetic in the right. The radiologist determined that my breasts were fibrocystic and that the lump appeared to be "probably benign." The doctor told me I had fibrocystic breast disease. I was just being paranoid after my surgery. And who wouldn't be after hearing about this new type of inflammatory breast cancer, which I will address. In **fibrocystic disease**, the breast duct becomes blocked and fills up with fluid; that is the cystic component of fibrocystic disease. The area around the blocked duct has a tendency to form scar tissue, and that's the fibrous component of the fibrocystic disease. The bad news is that they are painful, and there is no cure. Fibrocystic breasts are lumpy to begin with, but once a lump is found, as was the case with me, if it is not removed it has to be monitored every six months in case there is a change in that area. Many doctors believe that this condition is "normal." In women, however, medical and scientific studies not to mention the pain women experience, has shown that this disease is not so "normal" and that there is also an increased risk of breast cancer. Doctors have recommended eliminating caffeine and eating a high-fiber diet to reduce the level of pain.

As King Solomon said, "There is nothing new under the sun," and there is nothing new about **inflammatory breast disease**. It's just new to the public because it's now affecting a greater portion of the population. A friend of mine was orphaned because of the disease and left to raise her sisters, and she is now in her late forties. It is a type of breast cancer where the breast feels warm and looks red and swollen. The skin has the appearance of an orange. The redness warmth are caused by the cancer cells blocking the lymph vessels in the skin. The inflammatory portion of this disease is the nipple has inverted, as such resembling an orange.

This is an illustration of inflammatory breast cancer.

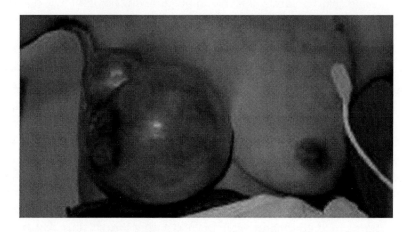

The following image is what breast cancer looks like. Do not wait! Have regular mammograms. It will save your life!

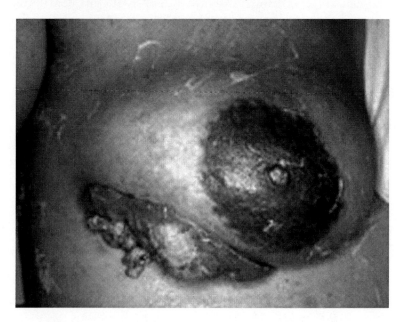

CHAPTER TWENTY-THREE

Tear-Left Rotator Cuff/Bursitis

It was the spring of 2003. There is nothing like a southern spring. There are flowers blooming everywhere and bumblebees the size of a golf ball. After having been born and raised in Queens, New York, I love seeing so many varieties of birds. You can even see hummingbirds drinking nectar from flowers. Looking out from my kitchen window, I can see chipmunks frolicking in my backyard. I remember one morning I was up early and went out on the deck and I saw a baby rabbit. When I looked in the direction that it ran, there was an opossum sitting on the fence. Spring is a time of renewal. At the time of the first writing this book, I have been living in Georgia eight years, and I am still mesmerized by the beauty of a southern spring. There are so many white and purple trees and majestic oaks in bloom. To me, the time was significant for change. I had had enough of this neurologist who was obviously unfamiliar with rare diseases and **didn't have a clue** what was wrong with me. I wanted, needed, a second opinion. I knew there was something wrong with my shoulder, neck, and spine, and I was tired of his dismissive, condescending attitude. After all, it was my dollar, and I was not getting what I was paying for. There was a neurosurgeon that was highly recommended by Piedmont Hospital as a top-notch neurosurgeon. After an initial consultation, I simply told him what I had been telling my neurologist all along that my neck, left shoulder, and back hurt. He ordered the following tests: MRI of the upper joint without contrast, CT of the cervical spine with contrast, and a cervical myelogram. All these exams were administered on March 3, 2003. Because of the nature of the final exam, I was admitted to the hospital. I had no idea that my life was about to change. This was indeed a beginning.

Bursitis

Bursitis is a common form of rheumatism. Rheumatism is any painful condition involving muscles, joints, or connective tissues. It comes from the Greek word *rheumatismos* that means a flowing of mucus. Did you ever wonder why your neck or muscles feel stiff and ache during a flu or severe cold? It is because there is the presence of infected mucus in the muscles, joints, or connective tissues that causes inflammation. The result of overstraining the muscles is called muscular rheumatism and, of course, it involves muscles and not joints. Other kinds of rheumatism cause fever known as rheumatic fever; others cause arthritis, which affects the bones and is referred to as rheumatoid arthritis. When there is an inflammation of the lubricating spaces near the shoulder and hip joints, it is called bursitis.

An MRI of the left shoulder revealed abnormal fluid in the subacromial bursa. The bursa is a small fluid-filled bag that acts as a lubricating surface for a muscle to move over a bone. As the result of overactivity of an arm, leg, or knee, irritation may occur at the joint; and fluid will fill in the joint, and become painful, and make it difficult to move. An MRI will reveal the presence of not only the lubricating fluid but the abnormal fluid as well. The abnormal fluid may represent reactive bursitis.

Rotator Cuff Tear

The most common symptom of a rotator cuff tear is pain. As I stated earlier, MRIs do not lie. It is a medical fact that it is often difficult for a patient to localize the pain to a specific area. As such, when trying to describe the pain, it only made sense that with generalized movement the pain was viewed as "shifting from left to right." But, of course, a neurologist would not know this, and an orthopedic surgeon would, or would he? There may be loss of motion for a complete tear, and for an incomplete tear there will be decreased strength. The rotator cuff is a **common cause of pain and disability**. There are four muscles and tendons that form a cuff over the shoulder, allowing the shoulder the rotate—as such, the name rotator cuff. This injury is common in middle-aged people, athletes, and it is the result of trauma or degeneration of the tendon. Is it a coincidence that prostaglandins act on connective tissue or may exacerbate a condition as well? A lifting injury may also be the culprit, such as overdoing housework or gardening, repetitive overhead activity such as the daily work of a construction worker. The reported symptoms are stiffness or partial or complete loss of motion. You may have difficulty with simple tasks such as combing your hair. A patient may report sudden or acute pain that "switches." The reason for this is the complication, as it is in my case, of the presence of osteo or rheumatoid arthritis's affecting the cervical spine, which will be apparent upon examination by a trained physician. For a partial tear, treatment options include steroid injections, anti-inflammatory medication, rest, and a sling. If the arm does not improve, then the orthopedic surgeon may recommend surgery.

PIEDMONT HOSPITAL

DUPLICATE   FINAL

Name: BROWN,STACEY PRICE   Location: DIS - ODC
DOB: 05/23/59 Age: 43Y Sex: F   MR#   P002124569
Ordered Date/Time: Acct#: P0308500872
Ck-In Date/Time: 03/26/03 1418

Deliver to
                                            Attend. Dr
                          1 st   Admit. Dr
                                            Ref. Dr:
                          GA 30060   Ord. Dr
                                            PCP

Chk-in # Exam   Desc   Ord Diag.
1306442 78107   MRI UPPER JOINT W/O CONTRAST*L719.41-JOINT PAIN-SHLDER

FINDINGS: MRI of the left shoulder is performed. There are no plain
films for correlation. An abnormality of the glenoid labrum is not
detected. There is abnormal fluid in the subacromial bursa. This is
fairly small in amount and may represent reactive bursitis. This can be
a secondary sign of rotator cuff tear however. There is abnormal signal
in the humeral head near the rotator cuff insertion site on all pulse
sequences. This is believed to be related to cystic erosion in the
region of the greater trochanter. There is abnormal signal in the distal
rotator cuff but this does not brighten with progressive T2-weighting
and therefore is nonspecific in nature. Retraction of the rotator cuff
is not seen.

IMPRESSION: There are multiple findings which are not specific. Plain
film correlation is recommended. There is at least tendinosis or partial
thickness tear of the rotator cuff, but a complete thickness tear cannot
be confidently diagnosed on the basis of this study alone. There are
secondary changes in the bone and a small reactive bursitis in the
subacromial bursa.

                      Read By:
                      Released B   MD
                      Date/Time Released: 03/26/03 2136

PR
03/26/03 2136

FINAL   Radiology Report

XXXXXXFINALXXXXXFINALXXXXXXXFINALREPORTXXXXXXXFINALXXXFINALXXXXXXXXXXXXXXXXXXX

The MRI revealed a partial thickness tear of the left rotator cuff. I was referred to an orthopedic surgeon at Piedmont Hospital. Piedmont is listed as one of the top 100 hospitals in the United States. He recommended a cortisone injection and not to repair the tear because of my multiple medical problems. He did not want to operate unless it was absolutely necessary.

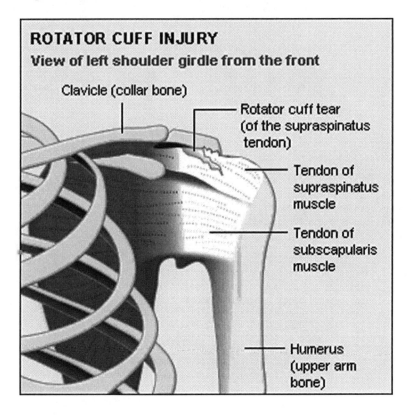

ROTATOR CUFF INJURY
View of left shoulder girdle from the front

Clavicle (collar bone)

Rotator cuff tear (of the supraspinatus tendon)

Tendon of supraspinatus muscle

Tendon of subscapularis muscle

Humerus (upper arm bone)

CHAPTER TWENTY-FOUR

Ossified Posterior Longitudinal Ligament Disease

In order to understand the diagnosis, we must first understand how the spinal column is designed. The spinal column or vertebral column supports the body. It is composed of a column of bones called vertebrae. There are thirty-three vertebrae altogether. They are held together by connective tissue called ligaments. In order to easily identify the parts of the spine, they have been broken into regions. The cervical

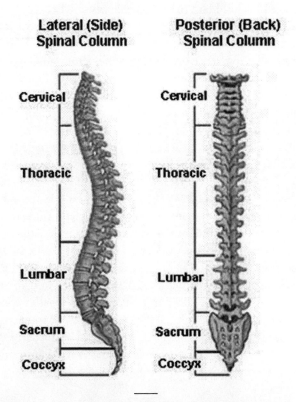

Lateral (Side) Spinal Column

- Cervical
- Thoracic
- Lumbar
- Sacrum
- Coccyx

Posterior (Back) Spinal Column

- Cervical
- Thoracic
- Lumbar
- Sacrum
- Coccyx

spine is composed of seven vertebrae and is located directly beneath the brain. In fact, the first cervical vertebra is called the atlas, and its job is to support the skull. On a radiology report, it would be referred to as C1. The next set of vertebrae is called thoracic. There are twelve altogether, and they are located in the chest region. The third set is composed of five vertebrae and are located in the lower back. They are referred to as the lumbar. The fourth set, referred to as the sacral, are fused together. The sacral are composed of five fused vertebrae, and they make up the hip region. The fifth and final section of the spinal column is called the coccyx. It is also composed of fused vertebrae; however, there are only four coccygeal or the tailbone.

Myelogram

The first of the tests was the cervical myelogram. After a local anesthetic was administered, the lumbar spine was punctured, and a contrast was injected to view the spine in a swimmer's position. I was literally strapped into position as the table began to tilt forward. I was not prepared for this. I felt as though I was going to slide off the table face first, and by the way I was strapped down, there was nothing I could do to brace myself if I came off the table. The technician reassured me I was safe. He must have had extrasensory perception because he told me I would not come off the table but that I had to keep absolutely still because there were needles sticking out my lumbar spine. As I felt the sensation of the contrast dye begin to warm and pulsate through my body, I began to slide forward. The realization that the needles were sticking out of my spine while simultaneously sliding forward was beginning to overwhelm me and I began to cry softly. The doctor continued to work and via microphone assured me that I was not going to fall. As the contrast continued pumping I felt the pressure and its presence creep through my body and make its way into my eyes, and I let out a yelp. He entered the room from the control room and asked what was wrong. I advised him of the foregoing, and he advised me that that had never happened before; however, I assured him that my eyes were on fire and my head felt as though it was about to burst. He just continued to reassure me that I was not going to fall off the table, that he had never lost a patient, and that I need not move especially since there were needles puncturing my spine. I tried to remain calm, but the tears began to well and flow both from fear and pain. I began to feel an underlying guilt that the radiologist had performed the myelogram as quickly as he could under the circumstances. Suddenly, I became aware of the fact that there was a technician in the room with me. He stood by, silently watching and changing film as he was ordered to do so by the radiologist. I lay there helplessly, praying for it to end quickly. I began to shake from the sudden awareness that I was cold and tired. I was asked to lie still, otherwise the test would have to be repeated. With that in mind, I complied. However, for the record, this is one painful, uncomfortable test.

Diagnosis

The test results identified very minimal scoliosis in the cervicothoracic region. This refers to the seventh vertebral disc and the first thoracic disc. It is also possible that these discs may be fused together resulting in a curve. Scoliosis is the curve or bend of a normally straight spine. It may be a single bend or multiple bends. The curves are usually in the form of an *S* or a *C*. It usually begins in childhood or early teens and can be corrected if detected early enough with proper treatment, which includes braces, exercise, or surgery. A paralyzed back muscle or a disturbance of growth—for example, a short leg—may account for this condition.

The neurosurgeon advised me that I had another rare disease, but this time it was of the spine. It was called ossified posterior longitudinal ligament disease. The diagnosis was a lot to take in, and the first place I went to was NORD for help. I realized how rare the disease was when they had no information in their databanks.

This is a disease commonly seen in Oriental people, especially people of Japanese descent. There is a strong genetic predisposition, and I was so desperate to find out what was wrong with me I even called Japan. Needless to say, they thought I was crazy; but they were polite, and I was right back where I started. The specialist I went to see was very charming. He started off our visit by saying, "You don't look Japanese." He urged me to look deeper into my family genetic history for answers, to perhaps explain the anomaly. It is possible to have this disease if you have abnormal calcium metabolism, a history of degenerative disc disease, ankylosing spondylitis, diffuse idiopathic skeletal hyperostosis or DISH, fluoride overdose, or diabetes mellitus. This disease usually affects men and involves the cervical spine but has been seen in the lumbar spine at the disc level, and onset is usually between fifty to seventy years old. Lesions of the posterior longitudinal ligament include hypertrophy, calcification, and ossification. Herniated disc material may deform the deep layer of the posterior longitudinal ligament, causing reactive fibrous proliferation and **inflammatory cellular changes,** resulting in severe cord compression. The treatment options are not attractive: simple laminectomy, expansive laminectomy, anterior spinal fusion, anterior cervical decompression consisting of discectomy, corpectomy, and resection of the OPLL mass. It seems I am destined to be the bride of Frankenstein after all, if this disease continues on its course.

The myelogram did not reveal nerve root sheath compression or cord compression, and a CT scan would have to be performed to evaluate these concerns. There was evidence of some bulging discs or possibly some thickening of the ligament flavum. This could be seen at multiple levels from C3 to C7. The ligaments are fibrous tissue, which hold together the vertebrae. They also hold organs of the body in place and fasten bones together. Ligaments are as strong as rope; however, they heal very slowly. When you hear the term *bulging disc*, you are referring to a ligament that is protruding between two vertebrae. Just picture a smore, if you will, and the ligament is the melted marshmallow. When you hear the term *degenerative disc*, then you are referring to a ligament that is tearing apart, or unraveling and not healing. When that happens, then the bones begin to rub together, resulting in unimaginable pain—like brakes without pads.

CT Scan

The CT scan of the cervical spine was the next exam that was performed. The exam confirmed asymmetric bulging on the right side at C3-C4 with compression of the dural sac ventrally. The dural sac is a tough fibrous membrane that covers the brain and spinal cord. In other words, ventral compression is on the lower surface of the vertebrae to the right side of C3 and C4. Ouch! However, there was no cord flattening, deformation, or nerve sheath compression identified. If this were the case, then paralysis would result. The spine is designed to communicate with the rest of body like a telecommunications center by the network of nerves. When the nerves stop communicating, then this causes paralysis. Paralysis means loss of muscle movement. There is a pair of nerves for each vertebra. The report went on to identify no evidence of foraminal stenosis. This is the condition that occurs when the opening in the vertebrae, which allows the nerves to pass, narrows. I have been diagnosed with cervical spondylosis. Foraminal stenosis is a disease process of cervical Spondylosis. Confirming diagnosis of the disease, the CT scan further reported thickening with "calcification in the posterior longitudinal ligament behind the vertebral bodies, starting at C3 and extending inferiorly." Calcification is the impregnation of tissue with calcium or calcium salts. The results are that the impregnated tissue will harden. As such the posterior longitudinal ligament, the one running lengthwise along the back of my neck, has calcified or is the process of doing so. The report confirms compression of the dural sac ventrally; however, it reveals further compression of the cervical spinal cord with flattening of the ventral aspect of the cord on the right behind the C3 vertebra. There is also thickening of longitudinal ligament with calcification on the right behind the L4 vertebral body, causing compression of the dural sac. When reference is made to L4, there is also cord compression and calcification in the lumbar region. This report confirms that I have the rare honor of having OPLL in both the cervical and lumbar regions—cord compression at both ends.

At C5-C6, the radiology report noted there is an "asymmetric extradural defect on the right which is soft tissue in nature, possibly associated with some posterior Osteophyte formation." An Osteophyte formation is a bony outgrowth that is occurring outside of the dural sac. We understand that the degenerative process is part of living, but please bear in mind that all these diseases are rare and that the average age for the completion of the process is sixty, and that most of them have been brought about by a breakdown in the inflammatory process of the human body gone haywire. Again, something set it off!

Again at C5 there is some calcification and thickening of the longitudinal ligament. As a result, it is causing compression on the right side of the cord behind the C5 vertebral body. At C5-C6 there is asymmetric focal bulging of the disc together with cord compression of the dural sac ventrally on the right side. As of March 2003, there was only minimal soft tissue thickening behind the C7 vertebral body, and there was no extradural defect noted from C7-T1 covering the rest of the spine.

Throughout the report it was noted in spite of the cord compression there was no nerve sheath compression. The nervous system of the human body is composed of the brain, the spinal cord, and the nerves, which extend throughout the body. The brain interprets the messages sent by the nerves as various sensations such as heat, pain, pleasure, light, smell, etc. The nerves are made up of cells that are called neurons. There are several billion neurons in the human body and each is connected with one another to form the nervous system. There are two different kinds of nerves. A nerve may be either a single neuron or a bundle of several nerves bound together by a tough sheet of tissue called a nerve trunk. A fat-containing myelin or medullary sheath covers this nerve trunk. The spinal cord is a long, thick nerve trunk that runs from the base of the brain down through the spinal column. The spinal cord is composed of white matter and gray matter. White matter is another name for the nerve fibers that are covered with white myelin sheath, and gray matter is the name given to the cell bodies and dendrites of neurons. A brief description of a nerve cell body is that it is called a neuron. The neuron is composed of a nucleus surrounded by a cytoplasm. The cytoplasm, which surrounds the nucleus, has at least one single thread called an axon, which can grow several feet. The axon then grows out into one or more fine branched threads called dendrites. The axon conducts impulses to the dendrite of another neuron or to an effector organ, such as a muscle cell. The spinal nerves, which come from the spinal cord, control the muscles of the body. There are eight pairs of cervical nerves in the first seven vertebrae of the spinal column. The next sets are twelve pairs of thoracic nerves, five pairs of lumbar nerves, five pairs of sacral nerves, and finally five pairs of coccygeal nerves at the base of the spinal column. These are part of the autonomic nervous system because they control activities that are involuntary or automatic, such as breathing and heart rate, and act independently of the central nervous system. These nerve fibers have no myelin sheath even though they are part of the peripheral nervous system. However, the central nervous system and the peripheral nervous system do contain myelin sheath. The central nervous system consists of the spinal cord and the four major divisions of the brain, as previously discussed. The peripheral nervous system consists of the twelve pairs of cranial nerves and thirty-one pairs of spinal nerves and the autonomic nervous system—although it is sometimes considered a separate system. Sensory nerves enter the spinal cord at the dorsal root. The motor nerves leave the spinal cord at the ventral root. If the ventral root is cut, then the part of the body to which the nerve leads cannot move, but it still has sensation. If the dorsal root is cut, sensation will disappear, but the body part can move. If there is myelin sheath compression ventrally or dorsally, then the body will act as though the nerve were cut.

The radiologist's impression of the CT scan was calcification of the posterior longitudinal ligament together with compression of the dural sac ventrally of the right side. Further, asymmetric bulging discs at C3-C4, C4-C5, C5-C6, and C6-C7 were postured to be the cause of the cervical spinal cord compression on the right of these levels.

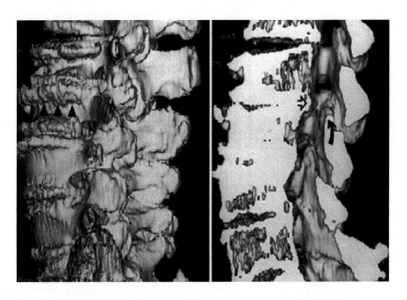

The Role of Prostaglandins in Ossified Posterior Longitudinal Ligament Disease

In the *Journal of Pharmacology and Experimental Therapeutics*,[1] first published on February 11, 2003, in an attempt to identify the genes that participate in OPLL it was discovered that a 283 base pair cDNA fragment corresponding to

---

[1] **Journal of Pharmacology and Experimental Therapeutics** *Fast Forward.* First published on February 11, 2003 by Hirotaka Ohishi, Ken Ichi-Furukawa, Koei Iwasaki, Kazumasa Ueyama, Seiko Harata and Satoshi Toh

the first receiver, GPCR, prostaglandinI2, does play a role in the gene expression induced by mechanical stress in spinal ligament cells derived from patients with ossification of the posterior longitudinal ligament of the spine. OPLL cannot occur without ectoptic bone formation in the spinal ligaments and mechanical stress. So let's start from the beginning. After taking Vioxx, a tumor developed at the base of the brain/cervical spine. Ectoptic bone formation is a bone—in my case, a chrondroma that formed outside of the spine. As previously indicated, this was a rare tumor. Exactly what is mechanical stress? Mechanical stress is a procedure such as laminectomy or laminoplasty, which causes **biological stimulation, defect of the dorsal element, and cervical instability**. There are many studies and clinical evidence that support the hypothesis that mechanical stress acts on the posterior ligaments and will lead to the progression of OPLL.

After many tests were conducted, it was concluded that prostaglandin receptors play a **major role** in the progression of OPLL. Although I did not have decompression surgery, OPLL was activated through **biological stimulation through the activation of the PGI2 signaling system, which affects the progression of OPLL.** PGI2 interacts with a specific receptor, IP, which is a G protein-coupled cell surface receptor or GPCR, the first receptor in the immune response. Scientists detected this IP receptor in fetal bone and osteoblasts. Osteoblasts are the cells that make up the framework of the bone, and osteoclasts are the cells that build new bone. PGI2 interacts with a specific receptor, IP. Ligament cells have been reported to express other prostaglandin receptors.

CHAPTER TWENTY-FIVE

Diffuse Idiopathic Skeletal Hyperostosis

Diffuse idiopathic skeletal hyperostosis is a disease associated with ossified posterior longitudinal ligament disease. It is considered a form of degenerative arthritis. The paraspinal ligaments degenerate second to attrition, and then ossify. In other words, calcification occurs along the sides of the vertebrae of the spine. There is excessive bone growth along the sides of the spine. This process is called spinal enthesopathy. Enthesopathy involves degenerative disorders. It is the abnormal attachment of a tendon or a ligament to a bone, and it involves an inflammatory process. Three conditions are associated with this phenomenon. Ossification of the vertebral arch ligaments or a condition called OVAL. Forestier's disease involves ossification of the anterior longitudinal ligament. OPLL involves the posterior longitudinal ligament and DISH has similarities between the two. Osteophytes will form in response to degenerative disc disease. DISH distinguishes itself because it usually affects the lower thoracic spine region, but it can also affect the lumbar and cervical spine. It causes bony changes in these areas called spurring. Patients with DISH suffer with stiffness and pain and a condition called kyphosis, which is an abnormal rearward curvature of the spine often confused by the **untrained** as "loss of lordosis." (I actually had a rheumatologist enter this in a report. Incidentally it was the same one who suggested the rehabilitation.) These aforementioned conditions are the results of the inflammation of the tendons and ligaments that attach to the bone. This will occur at the knee, the elbow, and the heel of the foot; and bone spurs may develop as a result. In my case, you can actually hear crepitus sounds when I move at the aforementioned locations. This condition is confused with tendonitis in that the symptoms are similar. Stiffness is worse in the morning or after long periods of sitting. Dry climates are preferable as wet weather will exacerbate this condition. Although this condition was noted in medical literature for approximately one hundred years, it was not recognized as a distinct medical condition until 1997.

DISH is rarely seen in African Americans, but guess who has it? If you said the author of this book, you were right. It is rare in persons under fifty, and it affects men more than women. DISH is the second most common form of arthritis after osteoarthritis. So let's review the symptoms of DISH. It is accompanied with back pain and stiffness, especially in the middle of the back; there are problems with swallowing and movement of the neck, and it is accompanied with what seems like tendonitis in the shoulder, elbow, knee, or ankle. The disease is usually confirmed by x-ray of the thoracic spine and chest, showing bony outgrowths of DISH along the vertebrae.

This following is an illustration of DISH. It illustrates bony outgrowths along the spine, together with calcification along the vertebrae.

Diffuse Idiopathic Skeletal Hyperostosis

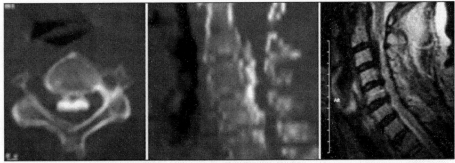

Fig 2. Cervical CT and MRI scans showing spinal cord compression due to OPLL.

CHAPTER TWENTY-SIX

Sciatica

Sciatica affects 3 percent of the population. As the name indicates, the pain runs along the sciatic nerve when the nerve is pinched and irritated. Pain may also result from a herniated disc. Sciatica usually affects one side of the lower body and will usually last for weeks or months, not requiring surgical intervention. For others pain can be more debilitating. Constant shooting pain, making it difficult to stand, burning or tingling down the leg, and nerve damage may result. In this instance, a lumbar laminectomy may be required to preserve nerve function and relieve inflammation. The pain may also be suddenly felt down the buttocks and to the back of one thigh and into the leg. When this occurs, a protruding disc in the spinal column is more than likely pressing down on the roots of the sciatic nerve. This is called lumbar radiculopathy. Pain may also be felt when coughing or sneezing. In some cases, patients experience leg cramps for weeks, pins and needles sensations, and weakness in the leg on one side. Onset is usually between the ages of thirty and fifty, and sciatica can easily be diagnosed through an MRI. In my case, it was difficult to determine what course of action to take because of the complications of a herniated disc together with multiple sclerosis, which produce the same symptoms: burning, tingling, etc.

Sciatica

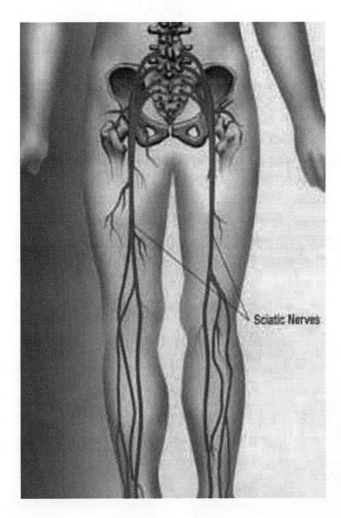

Piedmont Hospital Emergency Department
1968 Peachtree Rd. N.W., Atlanta, GA 30309
(404) 605-3297

Sciatica

Your exam shows you have sciatica, a condition most often seen in patients with disc disease of the lower back. Sciatica causes pain to radiate from the lower back or buttock area down the leg. It results from pressure on nerve roots coming out of the spine when a disc deteriorates and pushes to one side. Often there is a history of back problems. Sciatica symptoms are reported in about 3% of the population.

In most cases sciatica improves greatly with conservative treatment. Most patients with it are completely better after 2-4 weeks of bed rest and other supportive care. Bed rest reduces the disc pressure greatly; sitting is the worst position since the pressure on the disc is over 5 times greater than it is while lying down. You should avoid bending, lifting, and all other activities which make the problem worse. After the pain improves, you may continue with normal activity, taking brief periods for bed rest throughout the day until you are back to normal.

Aspirin, ibuprofen, or other anti-inflammatory drugs are often used to help control pain. Muscle relaxants may help by relieving spasm and providing mild sedation. Cold or heat therapy and massage may also give significant relief. Spinal manipulation is not recommended because it can increase the degree of disc protrusion. Traction can be used in severe cases. Surgery is reserved for patients that do not improve within the first months of conservative treatment, or who have signs of severe nerve root pressure.

You should see your doctor for follow up care as recommended. A program for back injury rehabilitation with stretching and strengthening exercises is an important part of management. Please call your doctor, a back specialist, or the emergency room right away if you notice increased pain, weakness, or numbness in your legs, or if you have any difficulty with bladder or bowel control.

CHAPTER TWENTY-SEVEN

Multiple Sclerosis

On April 18, 2003, I was driving my children to school. I had barely digested the news of these new rare spinal diseases when I found out the hard way that I had no peripheral vision. A car was approaching, and being a courteous driver, I moved over to the right; however when I did, I took out my neighbor's mailbox and my side-view mirror at the same time. My vision had suddenly failed. Not only had I damaged the mirror to the tune of four hundred dollars on a two-year old Ford Expedition, I was horrified because this had never happened before. I sat there stunned. My vision was suddenly blurred, and then I just couldn't see out of the right side of my eye. I had to get it together quickly because I didn't want to frighten my children any more than I already had. I regrouped, returned home, and told my husband what had just happened. I immediately went to Piedmont Hospital emergency room. The physician's assistant from the dermatologist's office joined us in the emergency room and had my records with her just in case the loss of vision was related to the T Cell lymphoma. The Lord truly broke the mold when he created her. She told my husband to take the children home, and she waited with me all day from 9:00 a.m. to 7:00 p.m. The emergency room doctor ordered an MRI. I had just had an MRI less than a month ago, and here I was back here again. When the doctor walked through the door, I was not prepared for what he had to tell me. I was still accepting the fact that I might have some rare blood abnormality. Less than a month ago, I had just learned of the rare diseases affecting my spine, which meant that my spine is compressed and degenerating, leading to possible paralysis and inevitable bride-of-Frankenstein syndrome (my phraseology). Now this doctor told me that the test results were positive for multiple sclerosis. *Have mercy, Jesus,* I snapped. I just couldn't bear any more. Multiple sclerosis! I pulled out the IV and cried out in disbelief. I repeated what I had just gone through in the past few months and cried out, "This can't be happening, not to me!" Through my blurred visual field of tears, I looked around the room and realized everyone had their heads hung low, wiping tears, or shaking their heads; and they just allowed me to absorb the shock because there was nothing I could do to change what was. I remained legally blind for three weeks.

Multiple sclerosis is an autoimmune disease. It is a chronic, often disabling, disease of the central nervous system. The central nervous system includes the nerves of the brain and the spinal cord. The disease affects mostly women, and each week averages of two hundred new cases diagnosed. It is estimated that there are 400,000 people in the United States living with multiple sclerosis as of 2005. Onset of this disease is usually between the age of twenty and fifty years old. Symptoms can range from blindness to numbness in the limbs to paralysis. The severity and specific symptoms of MS in any one person cannot be predicted while the disease is active. As in my case, the blindness reversed itself but left residual scarring on the brain. As previously discussed, once brain cells die they do not regenerate, and the effects of MS last a lifetime. The nervous system is nourished by blood vessels that carry oxygen and nutrients throughout the white matter. In MS, errant T Cells, which are the key components of the body's immune system, somehow leak out of the blood vessels and cause swelling and damage to the surrounding white tissue. These cells attack the myelin sheath of the nerve fibers. This process is called demyelination. When this happens, the nerves cannot send signals along the fibers. As such, people with MS will exhibit poor muscle coordination, numbness or tingling, weakness or fatigue. As I previously discussed, neurons are the cells that process information in the brain. The chemicals in the brain are called neurotransmitters, and they allow the neurons to communicate with each other. The disease itself is unpredictable. Your body is literally attacking itself. The multiple symptoms range from mild to severe: partial blindness, red-green color distortion (that's a good defense to use in court for a red light ticket—just kidding), burning sensations, tingling, prickling, pins and needles, numbness, paralysis, loss of sexual desire, depression, muscle weakness, impaired coordination and balance, difficulty walking and standing, slurred speech, dizziness, bowel and urinary complaints, tremors and jerking, difficulty concentrating, occasional hearing loss, memory loss—short term and long term are affected, attention and judgment are affected—shock sensations in the face and jaw.

On March 18, 2004, I experienced an unusual phenomenon. I was on my way to my new doctor, who is the director of the Multiple Sclerosis Center of Georgia. I was experiencing significant leg weakness, but I was determined to make my appointment and leave there and audition for Missy Elliot's new show. I was so excited. I told everyone in the waiting room and the staff I was going to blow her away. I even had a demo with me, and I was dressed to impress. The audition was only one exit away and I knew I had what it took to make it. As far as I knew there were no age limits, and being a singer, songwriter, petite, and a I knew I had pretty decent voice, and people always tell me I look a lot younger than

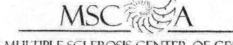

MSC A

THE MULTIPLE SCLEROSIS CENTER OF GEORGIA

WILLIAM H. STUART, M.D.   ROBERT W. GILBERT, JR., M.D.   ELLIS V. HEDAYA, M.D.
DOUGLAS S. STUART, M.D.   CHRISTOPHER S. RUSSELL, M.D.   JEFFREY B. ENGLISH, M.D.
ANDREI I. SERBANESCU, M.D.   LAWRENCE G. SEIDEN, M.D.
BEVERLY BAKER-NEWSHOLME, A.N.P., C.S.

March 18, 2004

Stacey P. Brown

Re: Cervical disc disease and myelopathy

To Whom It May Concern:

Stacey Brown, a patient of mine with multiple sclerosis, has a second neurologic problem which is the presence of a significant disc herniation at C-6, 7, with spinal cord effacement and pressure predominately on the right side as well as root foraminal encroachment.

She is in danger of significant cord compression and has been referred to a neurosurgeon for a second opinion with the probability that surgery will be required.

Her leg weakness which has been recently acquired is, I believe, due to this rather than multiple sclerosis. Her multiple sclerosis at the present time is stable. No additional change needs to be made in the treatment of that particular illness.

Sincerely,

William H. Stuart, M.D.

WHS:rb

I really am, I thought I had a chance. I told him of my desires, and I was quickly reduced to tears. He gently told me that my cord compression had significantly worsened and as a result it was causing my legs to become weak. The MRI revealed significant disc herniation at C6-C7, spinal cord effacement, pressure predominately on the right side together with root foraminal encroachment. He advised me to "hang up my dancing shoes." He prepared a letter dated March 18, 2004, for me to carry around with me addressed "To Whom It May Concern," to be presented to the neurosurgeon of my choice and to keep it with me, just in case. I had to face my reality that I have a disease that is affecting my T Cells. I also have a constant low white count and am dangerously anemic. All these rare diseases are wreaking havoc on my central nervous system, blood, and spine. Instead of heading to the audition, I was headed to the hospital for an MRI and for one of many neurosurgical consultations. The neurosurgeon advised that I would have to live with the leg weakness caused by the OPLL until such time as the disease process progressed into an unsteady gait, my handwriting would noticeably begin to change, I would have bowel and bladder dysfunction and significant cord compression before he would decompress my spine in order to relieve the leg weakness with a series of pins and screws strategically placed along the cervical and lumbar spine.

How would one categorize multiple sclerosis? It is categorized as an inflammatory disease of the central nervous system. As such, we can understand how prostaglandins are involved in the disease process of multiple sclerosis. In order to understand the inflammatory response, we must first understand the immune response. T cells are white blood cells, and as such, they are a part of your immune system. Their job is to fight bacteria and viruses as they enter the body. T cells are called leukocytes and are part of the immune system called the acquired immune system. The reason it is referred to as acquired is because as individual as we are, each person's immune system is unique, and as such it adapts to their specific needs. The features of an individual's immune system are learned during their lifetime in order to fight bacteria and viruses as they are exposed to them. This type of immunity begins in the bone marrow with a type of white cell or lymphocyte called a B cell or basophil. Their specific job is to attack a bacterium, which is identified as a foreign invader as it enters the body, destroy it, and build up a natural or acquired immunity. B cells, as previously discussed, originate in the bone marrow. These B cells mature in an organ called the thymus. Once these cells have matured, they are called lymphocytes. Lymphocytes have receptors on the cell surface that recognize broken-down protein fragments called antigens. When a lymphocyte and an antigen bind together, an immunological response will occur, and the body will defend itself. An autoantigen appears when the body "tags" its own tissue and begins to destroy it. This is referred to as an autoimmune disease, such as multiple sclerosis, and there is no pathogen involved.

The nerves of the human body are insulated with myelin. Myelin is composed of lipids, which are composed of fatty acids and proteins. Steroids are a class of lipids, and we should be aware there are a wide range of steroids. There is a difference between natural and synthetic steroids and anabolic steroids. All steroids, depending on the dosage and duration of use, can have serious side effects including high blood pressure, unwanted hair growth, swelling, menstrual cycle disruption, and even death. They are commonly used in the treatment of multiple sclerosis and to build up strength and muscle in seriously ill patients. In living organisms, lipids are the fuel tanks of cell membranes. When a nerve is covered or sheathed, it will receive an impulse or information at a greater speed than a nerve that is not covered or sheathed. This is the reason it is called a myelin sheath. The disease process of multiple sclerosis **destroys** the coating or sheath over the nerve fiber and decreases the signal. So the best example that I can give you is the Verizon Wireless commercial. Once the nerve sheath is destroyed or removed, how it acts on your brain, muscles, and every other part of your body that is affected. It's like, *Can you hear me, feel me, sense me, touch me, and see me now?* Nerve pulses that once transmitted from 5 to 30 meters per second are now decreased to 0.5 to 2 meters per second. Myelin is part of your central and peripheral nervous systems, and the process is called demyelination. That is why multiple sclerosis is called the demyelination disease.

When a multiple sclerosis patient suffers an attack anywhere in the body, steroids are the first line of defense. Steroids can make the difference between a patient being able to see, walk, feel, and breathe, or any of the basic functions that we take for granted that we are able to do on a daily basis. When a patient experiences a sudden relapse, any part of the body can suddenly stop working normally. There is no time frame as to when it will return to normal or *if* it will return to normal; and that is the scary part about the disease. Scientists have discovered that animal and human ovaries produce peptide hormones. The most potent compounds were found in mammals. They found that synthesizing the ovaries of these mammals produced a medical benefit As a result, today we have various steroid compounds including female oral contraceptives, estrogen replacement therapy, and the greatest benefit is with multiple sclerosis patients. The electrical signals are interrupted because of the process of the disease. Steroids act as a coating over the nerve that has been exposed due to the disease process. Anabolic steroids, on other hand, are man-made. In other words, they were produced by scientists in a laboratory. They are chemicals; and because they are chemically based, once ingested, the side effects are liver and kidney tumors, cancer, body trembling, liver damage, aggression and psychiatric side effects including manic episodes leading to violence.

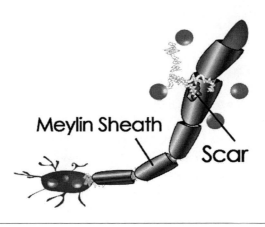

Meylin Sheath

Scar

PIEDMONT HOSPITAL

DUPLICATE   FINAL

Name: BROWN,STACEY PRICE
DOB: 05/23/59 Age: 44Y Sex: F
Ordered Date/Time:
Ck-In Date/Time: 03/10/04 1647

Location: DIS - ODC
MR# : P002124569
Acct#: P0407000968

Deliver to:

Attend
Admit
Ref.
Ord.
PCP:

ATLANTA   GA 30309

- -

Chk-in # Exam   Desc   Ord. Diag.
1604310 78068 MRI BRAIN W/WO   723.1-CERVICALGIA

TECHNIQUE: Sagittal T1, axial PD, T2, T1 pre- and post-contrast, and
coronal post-contrast images. Axial and sagittal FLAIR sequences and
coronal post-contrast images were obtained.

COMPARISON: 4/18/03

CLINICAL HISTORY: MS and history of T-cell lymphoma.

FINDINGS: Images demonstrate multiple foci of hyperintense signal
changes noted predominantly but not limited to the periventricular white
matter. Several of these oriented with their long axis perpendicular to
the long axis of the lateral ventricles. These are best seen on FLAIR
sequences. The hyperintense changes are stable when compared to the
previous exam. No enhancing lesions are noted. These findings are
compatible with the demyelinating process and a diagnosis of MS. The
lesions are only seen in the supratentorial area. There is questionable
enhancement of an area in the left centrum semiovale. There is also a
very faint area of enhancement noted in the lesion in the right temporal
horn. This lesion is new when compared to the previous exam. There are
two new lesions noted in the left frontal region.

IMPRESSION:

Findings compatible with diagnosis of MS with multiple hyperintense
changes in the supratentorial white matter. There is one focus of
enhancement noted adjacent to the right temporal horn which is new.

FINAL   CONTINUED Radiology Report

XXXXXXFINALXXXXXFINALXXXXXXXFINALREPORTXXXXXXFINALXXXFINAXXXXXXXXXXXXXXXXXX

DUPLICATE   FINAL

Name: BROWN,STACEY PRIC...   Location: DIS - ODC
DOB: 05/23/59   Age: 44Y Sex: F   MR#   P002124569
Ordered Date/Time: Acct#: P0407000968
Ck-In Date/Time: 03/10/04 1647

Deliver to   Attend. Dr:
          1   Admit. Dr.
                                     Ref.
          ATLANTA   GA 30309 Ord.
                                     PCP:

Checkin-Exam Code Summary
1604310-78068

   There appear to be two new lesions in the left centrum semiovale. No
   other findings. No mass effect.
                         Read By: LC
                         Released By:
                         Date/Time Released: 03/11/04 1544

AC
03/11/04 0841

FINAL   Radiology Report

XXXXXXFINALXXXXXFINALXXXXXXXFINALREPORTXXXXXXFINALXXXFINALXXXXXXXXXXXXXXXXXXX

The talk show host Montel Williams suffers MS, and he wanted to take his life. He wrote a book about it, *Climbing Higher*, and was featured in an article, "Back from the Brink" in the January 19, 2004, issue of *People* magazine. He reveals how MS drove him to attempt suicide. I read that article, thinking, *Here I am with all these diseases including MS. I now jerk at night because of MS. I don't have the financial security that he has. I have three children and a husband that are depending on me and are watching me in chronic pain on a daily basis.* Somewhere in the back of your mind, you are constantly thinking about waking

This is an illustration of the peripheral and central nervous systems of the human body—everything that is affected by multiple sclerosis.

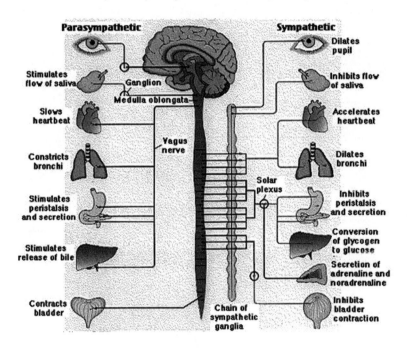

up one day and not being able to walk; and, believe me, that thought alone is frightening. Your body is slowly shutting down. I was diagnosed with what is called relapsing-remitting. One minute I have it and the next I don't. My children watched me roll down the hill and hit my head on the car parked at the bottom the hill outside of our home after picking them up from school when my legs collapsed from underneath me. There is never any warning. The attacks may last anywhere from minutes to weeks to months to permanent. How dare he even think about taking a life so precious that God gave him? We have to deal with the hand that we were given. With Jesus there is peace. Montel advocates using medical marijuana to treat MS. Some swear by medical marijuana, but I don't believe they made an informed decision especially when it comes to using it to treat multiple sclerosis. Their argument is simply that marijuana is natural. I am going to try to shed some light on what marijuana is. For me, it was never an option.

At first my doctor recommended no treatment, but because of the tremendous stress, that I was under I had to begin taking Avonex. When I saw the length of the needle, I literally cried. I measured the needle while it was still inside the sterile packaging, and it measures almost two inches. The needle has to be completely inserted into the thigh muscle once a week, alternating injection sites from the left to the right side of the body. When I first began my treatment, the Avonex Corporation sent out a nurse to show me how to inject myself. The treatment is very expensive. They followed up with a call the next week to see if I was successful and injected without difficulty. Sticking a two-inch needle in your leg is difficult. My daughter was nine years old when I first began injecting and wants to be a neurosurgeon. She volunteered to be my coach. I am very proud of her. When I can't bring myself to inject she says, "Mommy, the needle or the wheelchair," and with that sentiment, the needle goes in. I started jerking when I try to rest and a burning sensation started in my legs and has continued for almost two years. Sometimes the burning is unbearable, but it wasn't enough to concern my doctor because these are normal complaints with MS patients. With my multiple diagnoses, it may be the sciatica causing the burning. I have blurred vision from time to time, and the heat affects me. As my children put it, "Mommy is acting crazy," because I get very agitated out of fear of the side affects, which include death, if I am exposed to heat too long; and I am very serious about "cooling down." There was a news article on Monday, June 27, 2005, that an Ohio woman with MS died from sunbathing. I love the beach and swimming.

I quickly learned about heat and the side effects of multiple sclerosis. I volunteered to read for my daughter's fifth-grade class. There is never any warning. The symptoms will come on suddenly. It was the end of the school year, May 2005. I also write children's books and poetry, and in the middle of reading to them my eyes began to blur, my speech began to slur, my legs got weak, and my right leg became weak and started dragging. I was *so* embarrassed. My daughter looked at me and gave me that all-knowing look. She knew I was having an attack. Thank God for her. I was more concerned for her than for myself because you know how children are. If there was a hole I would have jumped into it. I just took a deep breath and kept going. What made it worse is the children probably thought I was drunk or on drugs because they are all part of a drug awareness campaign called DARE. I will never forget how her teacher looked at me. I know their parents got an earful that afternoon.

Ohio Woman With MS Dies From Sunbathing

By Associated Press

Mon Jun 27, 10:26 PM

WATERVILLE, Ohio - A woman with multiple sclerosis who sunbathed several hours in 95-degree heat at her nursing home in northwestern Ohio apparently died of a fever, which measured 109 degrees, the coroner's office said Monday.

Patricia Matney, 49, could walk only with assistance because of the disease and was on a blanket on a patio at the facility, said Steve Kahle, a Lucas County coroner's investigator.

Staff members at the Heartland of Browning nursing home periodically checked on her before she was found unconscious Sunday afternoon. Matney regularly spent time outdoors at the facility, said Julie Beckert, communications director for owner HCR Manor Care.

People with multiple sclerosis are particularly susceptible to heat because slight body temperature changes can aggravate symptoms of the nervous system disease, such as speech defects and loss of muscle coordination and eyesight, said Kottil Rammohan, an associate professor of neurology at Ohio State University.

Rammohan said he warns patients not to spend much time in saunas or whirlpools and advises them never to sunbathe alone.

When I first started my multiple sclerosis treatment, I asked the Avonex people what is Avonex made of? Jokingly I postulated, dehydrated monkey brains? I really expected the person on the other end of the phone to laugh, but I was asked to hold. After a long silence, someone returned to the phone, repeated my question, and answered, "No, it's actually made up of the ovaries of the female Chinese hamster." Perhaps that is why Montel will only put natural things in his body like medical marijuana if dehydrated female Chinese hamster eggs are the alternative. I try not to think about what I am injecting, but the "natural" alternative is not so natural and marijuana actually contains over **four hundred chemicals** not to mention the other pesticides used by whoever grew the plants. Marijuana has side affects that I do not believe marijuana smokers are fully aware of.

Medical Marijuana

The marijuana plant, as it is commonly known, dates back thousands of years and is believed to be a native plant of India where it originated in a region north of the Himalayan Mountains. The scientific name for the plant is *Cannabis sativa*. The plant can grow in height anywhere from thirteen to eighteen feet, and its flowers bloom from late-summer to mid-fall. The flowers that the plant produces are known as male and female and are differentiated by their appearance; male flowers are elongated and turn yellow and female flowers are spiderlike clusters and remain dark green. Hashish is what is made from the resin of the cannabis flowers and is much more powerful than marijuana. Again, most people are unaware of the fact that marijuana contains four hundred chemicals, sixty of which are cannabinoids. A cannabinoid is the major active ingredient in cannabis medicines, and THC is the chemical most often associated with the affects that marijuana has on the brain. The concentration of THC and other cannabinoids varies and depends on genetics and processing after harvest. THC stands for delta-9-tetrahydrocannibinol, which is the plant's main psychoactive chemical. Marijuana contains the same cancer-causing chemicals as cigarettes; it affects the brain's short-term memory, it increases the heart rate and raises levels of anxiety and **affects muscle coordination**. As a multiple sclerosis patient, it begs the question, why would you want to use a substance that affects your muscle coordination and short-term memory when the disease already does that?

This is a picture a marijuana leaf.

This is marijuana ready to be smoked or consumed.

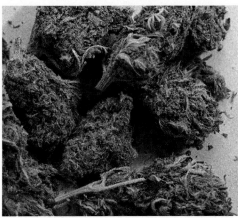

A study conducted by the National Multiple Sclerosis Society with ten individuals participating showed that marijuana use decreased muscle coordination. Marijuana smokers describe feeling relaxed and mellow immediately after smoking. Here's why. In your brain, there are groups of cannabinoid receptors concentrated in several places. Remember the neurons I previously discussed? Some neurons have thousands of receptors that are specific to its neurotransmitters and foreign chemicals like THC can mimic or block and then interfere with normal brain function. In the brain there are groups of cannabinoid receptors activated by a neurotransmitter called anandamide. THC is also a receptor. When you smoke marijuana it mimics or blocks the neurotransmitter anandamide and begins to act on the three cannabinoid receptor sites in the brain: the basal ganglia, hippocampus and the cerebellum. The hippocampus interferes with the recollection of recent events or short-term memory; the basal ganglia is responsible for unconscious muscle movement and the cerebellum controls coordination. Some go further to say that they don't smoke it, they ingest it in food. When marijuana is eaten, the stomach breaks it down; the blood absorbs it there and carries it to the liver and the rest of the body. The THC levels are lower, but the effects last longer. So my question is this, would a person who suffers from multiple sclerosis now armed with this information still make a conscious decision to smoke or ingest medical marijuana? Knowing the debilitating effects of the disease, I really don't think there are many options. Your physician doesn't warn you about the many side effects of the disease and the onset is sudden weakness of strength in your legs and muscles, extreme fatigue, shocks in your face and hands, burning sensation, muscle pain, bone pain, trouble with simple word recall, and in my own personal experience people are **not nice or sympathetic to your plight at all especially when you start stuttering.** As my pastor would say, "Be victorious and not a victim."

CHAPTER TWENTY-EIGHT

Hematuria

Hematuria is the abnormal excretion of red blood cells in the urine and is a sign that something is causing bleeding in the genitourinary tract. The indications are different for a man and a woman. For a man, doctors would be concerned that there would be prostate gland involvement, and for a woman viral infections of the urinary tract or a sexually transmitted disease. On August 9, 2003, I had difficulty urinating. There was a little straining, but there was nothing significant to report. By the time I got home from the rheumatologist, I was going to the bathroom every ten minutes. Frequent urination was one thing but then the unthinkable happened; when I went to the bathroom this time, there was an unusual straining accompanied by pain! When I looked, there was blood and mucous in the toilet. This is called gross hematuria because the blood is visible to the naked eye. Naturally, I had cause to be concerned. I arrived at the emergency room at three in the morning. Of course, by the time I got there, my urine was clear. I was hoping the doctors didn't think I was crazy. Although my urine was clear, the test was positive: Hematuria, blood in the urine. Mine was called microscopic hematuria. A CT scan of my kidneys was immediately ordered. The urinalysis ordered by the rheumatologist that morning showed no signs of infection or bacteria so I just assumed this would pass, excuse the pun. The tests noted only a few mucous threads and were negative for the presence of bacteria and infection. The CT scan was also negative and noted no kidney stones or tumors. These test results were unusual due to the absence of infection, bacteria, or stones. As a Band-Aid, antibiotics were ordered. I contacted my primary care physician the next morning. I was immediately referred to a urologist. Perhaps I made a poor decision that day, but I never kept that appointment. I had reached my breaking point after having been treated so poorly by that rheumatologist and his staff. I just couldn't bear anymore.

The genitourinary tract consists of the kidneys and tubes that carry the urine out of the body. Bleeding may only happen once as it did with me or it may be recurrent. Only 10 percent of the population experience hematuria. It is caused by kidney and bladder stones, medication such as Vioxx, trauma, urinary tract blockage, viral infections, and sexually transmitted diseases, prostate, and kidney disease. Since everything else had been ruled out, the only thing that could be ruled in would be the next set of things to be considered: rare diseases and genetic disorders. Hematuria will result from disorders such as sickle cell anemia or lupus, which is a chronic inflammatory disorder of the connective tissue. I had already been tested for lupus and sickle cell anemia, and the results came in negative. In my case, the hematuria was probably caused by the combination of the onset of so many autoimmune disorders. But we will never know.

for STACEY BROWN, Sunday, August 10, 2003, 3:41 am
(#0557091 Birthdate: 05/23/1959)

Our goal is to provide you OUTSTANDING treatment in a safe
environment. If for any reason you consider our care less
than outstanding, please contact the Emergency Department
Director so that we can provide better service in the
future.

IMPORTANT: We have examined and treated you today on an
emergency basis only. This is not a substitute for, or an
effort to provide, complete medical care. It is impossible
to recognize and treat all injuries or illnesses in a single
Emergency Department visit. You must let your doctor check
you again. Tell your doctor about any new or lasting
problems. If you had special tests such as EKG's and X-rays,
we will review them again within 24 hours. We will call you
if there are any new suggestions. After leaving, you should
FOLLOW THE INSTRUCTIONS BELOW.

You were treated today by
Our jo..

TODAY YOUR DIAGNOSIS IS: HEMATURIA
than c

Do the following:
FOLLOW UP AND TAKE MEDICATIONS AS DIRECTED

Call your doctor if you have:
- any new or severe symptoms.

Fluids/Rest/Return
Increase fluids (Powerade/Gatorade), get plenty of rest,
and return to the Emergency Department for any worsening
conditions.

TRIMETHAPRIM & SULFA (Septra DS, Bactrim DS).
This is a mixture of two antibiotic medicines. That means
it fights infections caused by bacteria. It is quite safe.
You may have some side effects, including stomach ache and
diarrhea. Some people are allergic to sulfa. Allergy would
show up as **rash or itching, wheezing or shortness of breath.**
If you have severe or new symptoms or any signs of allergy,
CALL YOUR DOCTOR RIGHT AWAY.

Take this medicine until gone in the following dose: 1
tablet two times daily .

****
THESE ARE YOUR FOLLOW-UP INSTRUCTIONS!
****
Call within 48 hours to make an appointment to see Dr. Rabin
in 3 TO 5 DAYS. Be sure to tell them you were referred by
the E.R. You can reach t (7 237 Upper

CHAPTER TWENTY-NINE

Leiomyoma (Uterine Fibroid)/Hysterectomy

As I became a statistic, I found that there is something wrong; and we, as women, are too complacent and accepting. The questions to be asked is why are there so many women "needing" hysterectomies? Why are there so many of us with fibroid tumors and/or cysts and uncontrolled bleeding and endometriosis? Scientifically, there is no contributing factor that gives rise to who gets fibroids and who doesn't. When a woman decides to start her family and the older a woman waits to start having children, the higher there are other risk factors such as birth defects. Generally, fibroids were seen when a woman reached thirty to forty years, but the rules have changed and there is no medical answer. Generally, a uterine fibroid is a benign tumor that, as its name suggests, grows in the uterus of a women. It affects more than 30 percent of women, and the medical term is leiomyoma. As such the names *uterine myoma* and *uterine fibroid* are used interchangeably. Most of the time you will not know a fibroid is present, and it does not interfere with a women's body function until they begin to grow. When they begin to grow, they grow rapidly and can interfere with fertility; they can cause abnormal bleeding and pressure and pain on the bladder and in some rare cases the spine. Doctors have found there is some role between fibroid growth and estrogen. They grow quickly during pregnancy and have been shown to shrink during menopause. No one is sure why fibroid tumors develop. Although many prefer natural remedies as opposed to surgery, there is an herbal remedy for reducing fibroids without having to resort to surgery, but it only has been proven to work with small fibroids and should not be used during pregnancy or lactation. The remedy is called chaste tree berry also known as *Vitex (Vitex agnuscastus)*. Claims have been made that this natural tea has been shown to lower excess estrogen levels, but has not been endorsed by the FDA. As previously stated, tumors grow silently, and before you realize it, they have already grown to a size that this natural tea will have no effect on.

There are six different types of fibroid tumors. I have had the distinct displeasure of becoming intimately familiar with complications from fibroid tumors. I gave birth to my first child at the age of thirty-one and my last at the age of thirty-six. Some would say I was late starting my family, but I truly believe in being prepared to handle children before having them; I do digress.

Fibroids are classified by where they are located. Fibroids that are located inside the cavity of the uterus are called **intracavitary**. They usually cause bleeding and cramping between periods. Another type of fibroid can also grow partially in the cavity and just below the lining of the uterus also interfering with the menstrual process and causing pain and irregular bleeding. This type of fibroid is called a **submucous** fibroid, and the type of irregular bleeding and pain between the menstrual cycles that both types of these fibroids cause is referred

This is a picture of *Vitex* or chaste berry.

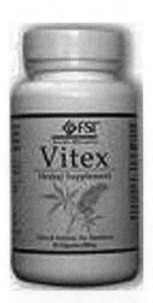 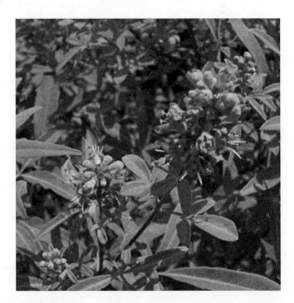

to as metrorrhagia. The third type of fibroid grows within the uterine wall and causes the uterus to enlarge as it grows and is called an **intramural** fibroid. The fourth type is called a **subserous** fibroid, and it grows on the outer wall of the uterus. A subserous fibroid can grow larger and begin to form a stalk and twist. As they grow, stalk and twist, they cause severe pain and connect themselves to the uterus by a stalk, which is very painful. When this occurs it is referred to as a **pedunculated** fibroid. The fifth type of fibroid is called an **intramural Myoma** because it grows in the wall of the uterus and can grow larger than a grapefruit. Rarely a fibroid can grow sideways between the ligaments, which support the abdominal region and the uterus. This type of fibroid is difficult to remove because it interferes with the blood supply of other organs. This is called an **interligamentous** fibroid.

I gave birth to two out of three children without incident. I began to have problems during and after the birth of baby Stacey. She was born after thirty-seven weeks, and there were no signs of fibroids in my uterus at the time; but my pregnancy was complicated due to other medical problems, and I almost lost her. Shortly after she was born, I began to have circulatory problems, as previously discussed. My menstrual cycle became longer and more painful, and my abdomen seemed to hurt all the time. Incidentally, I gave birth to my daughter in 1995, I took Vioxx in 1999, and my problems began in 2000. The uterine tumors formed and can be documented in 2002. I complained of pelvic pain, bleeding between periods, and heavy periods. My doctor performed a saline infusion sonogram on September 30, 2003, which allowed her to see the uterus clearly. The results were as follows: intracavitary fibroids, intramural fibroids, subserous and pendunculated fibroids, nabothian cyst on the cervix, endometriosis, and enlarged uterus. My doctor advised me that there were so many fibroids they could not be counted and that a hysterectomy would be my only option. She went on to say that I didn't need my uterus anyway! Wrong! My uterus was not some throw-away disposable product. God put it in there, and unless there was some alien abduction, it was staying in there. As such I adamantly objected to the surgical procedure, and I wanted a second opinion. In the meantime, my doctor suggested that I try medication: birth control pills, from the sixth through the fifteenth of each month to regulate my menses. The medicine was administered in low doses of estrogen, 10 mg each. I can only assume that my problem had already gone too far because my menses was now going from eight to twelve days at a time. The medicine was just not working, and the pain was getting worse. Often heavy bleeding is controlled with birth control pills, and in some cases it will decrease the size of the tumor; however, the effect is only temporary, and the fibroid will grow back to their pretreatment size once the medication is discontinued. I don't know why I thought the second opinion would be any different from the first. He also told me what I did not want to hear—a hysterectomy immediately. So I changed doctors again, hoping to change the outcome.

Nabothian cysts are cysts that can be found on the outside of the cervix. They look like small bumps and occur after new tissue grows after childbirth. These cysts are considered to be normal. They are filled with amber-colored mucus and can range in size from two to ten millimeters in diameter and usually are harmless unless they grow larger than ten millimeters. If that happens, then the fluid contained therein is tested for cancer cells. This can be easily detected with a routine examination.

Endometriosis

Researchers are beginning to find a link between autoimmune diseases and endometriosis. Endometriosis is a truly painful disease. The tissue that lines the uterus and is designed to nourish a newly fertilized egg will grow outside of the uterus and remain inside a woman's body, except that it will be found in the most unexpected places. In my case, my endometrial lining thickened to eight millimeters. The lining will shed at the time of menses, and attach itself to the bladder, bowel, vagina, and ligaments supporting the uterus or other parts of a woman's body, and then will constrict whatever it attaches itself to. In my case it also adhered to the ovaries, fallopian tubes, and other pelvic structures and caused lesions and scarring. I can only speculate as to the other parts of my body

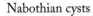

Nabothian cysts

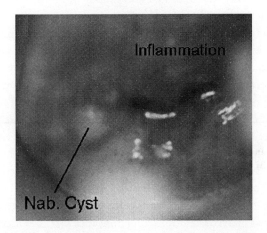

given all the autoimmune diseases that I now have. Patches of endometriosis may bleed during or in between the menstrual period, or the blood may build up and form cysts. Endometrial tissue continues to build up on itself each month and responds to the hormones of a woman's menstrual cycle, actually causing the endometriosis to increase each month, although the tissue breaks down and bleeds each month.

A woman's uterus is pear shaped and is held in place by several ligaments. The normal size is about the same as your fist. After fibroids begin to grow, they develop their own blood supply. They will continue to grow unless that supply is cut off. After many months of avoidance, the pain and bleeding were unbearable and I sought a third opinion. This doctor knew that I was afraid and that I did not want to have a hysterectomy. His advice to me was simply this: "When you are ready, let me know. And, in the meantime, I will make you as comfortable as I can." I just wanted to reach out and hug him. I knew I found the right doctor. He wasn't pushing surgery; he was leaving the decision to me although he advised me that hysterectomy would ultimately be a decision that I would have to consider. Office manner is **everything,** and I was making an informed decision without pressure, at least he led me to believe that I was making that decision.

My birth control method of choice was the IUD. One morning, during heavy menses, the cramping and pain were so unbearable I thought I was giving birth. The IUD was expelled; I was literally floored from the pain and crawled to the phone. My son had to pick me off of the floor. After explaining what had just happened between sobs to my gynecologist's office, I was begging them to set up a surgical date. They scheduled an emergency appointment. That is when my surgical options were first discussed.

Uterine artery embolization was not one of them. In light of my medical history, this procedure was not recommended, although my doctor advised me that it was, again, up to me. It is the process by which, under local anesthesia, a catheter is inserted into the femoral artery through an incision in the groin. Fibroids depend on a blood supply to grow. If that blood supply is cut off then the tumor will starve and shrink. There are two main blood supplies leading into the uterus. If that blood supply is blocked, then the theory is the tumors cannot survive. These arteries are blocked by plastic polyvinyl alcohol particles (PVA), which remain permanently in the vessels supplying the tumor. Over time the fibroids shrink; however, the procedure is usually performed by radiologists and not doctors. The problem with this procedure is that it is not reliable, and there were too many risks such as tumor expulsion, foul vaginal odor, severe pain and hematoma at the incision site, allergic reaction to the contrast material, infertility, vaginal discharge, continued tumor growth, menopause, and loss of orgasm. With all these risks, I felt my chances were better with a hysterectomy.

Another alternative procedure is called a **myomectomy**. It is the surgical removal of fibroids from the uterus without removing the uterus. There are actually three types of myomectomy procedures: (1) abdominal, which speaks for itself; (2) hysteroscopy, which is the insertion of a hysteroscope through the cervix into the uterus; and (3) laparoscopy, where several small incisions are made as opposed to one large incision. These procedures are based on where the fibroids are located and are performed if a woman wants to keep her uterus and continue having children. In my case, a myomectomy was out of the question because the wall of my uterus was 8 mm thick. This condition is called adenomyosis and is often confused with fibroids. In adenomyosis, the lining of the uterus infiltrates the wall of the uterus, causing it to thicken and enlarge. The same risks occur with the myomectomy as with the other procedures, and that is the risk that new fibroids can form and the ones left behind can continue to grow.

A hysterectomy has now become the second most common surgery among women in the United States. Over 80 percent of women between the ages of thirty to fifty years old have fibroids, although they only cause symptoms in 25 percent of these women. Of these women 50 percent to 75 percent are African American, and these women are 100 percent symptomatic. These statistics are staggering. Should we not be questioning what is now becoming a "natural" part of our adult lives? Genetics may play a role, but is it the real culprit? Is it diet or other environmental factors at work? Fibroids can begin to grow soon after puberty although they are not detected until a women reaches young adulthood. Risk factors for fibroids include being overweight, sedentary, early onset of menses before twelve years, and never being pregnant, or perhaps delayed childbirth.

People are under the misconception that there is one type of surgery for hysterectomy. When I discussed what I had been through with a "doctor" this person advised me to sue for malpractice because I still had my cervix. It was then that I realized that how much we don't know and understand about what is now becoming a basic procedure in our society. A **complete** or **total hysterectomy** removes the cervix as well as the uterus. This is the most common type of hysterectomy, although it is not always performed as was the case with me. A **partial** or **subtotal hysterectomy** removes the upper part of the uterus and leaves the cervix in place. A **radical hysterectomy** removes the uterus, cervix, and upper part of the vagina. What is removed is at the discretion of the surgeon. A radical hysterectomy will be performed where cancer is confirmed or suspected. The surgeon may also opt to remove the ovaries and fallopian tubes, resulting in the onset of menopause and can result in symptoms more severe than the natural onset of menopause. This procedure is called a **bilateral salpingo-oophorectomy**. A hysterectomy is performed by cutting through the abdomen or the vagina. In my case, I had what was called a **double hysterectomy**. In other words, the surgery was performed by cutting through the abdomen and the vagina because of the size of the uterus and the amount of myomas, which could only be removed from both ends. It was discussed before the surgery that my vagina, ovaries, fallopian tubes, and cervix would remain intact. The surgery went well; all things considered, however, the recovery period for a hysterectomy is approximately six weeks, and bleeding will vary, of course, depending upon the individual. I was very surprised that my heaviest bleeding was immediately following the surgery and did not continue when I got home, so I wasted those heavy pads because I hardly bled at all. I was just in pain and uncomfortable, for lack of a better word. I followed the doctor's instructions to the letter, much to my husband's chagrin, and thank God I did because by the third week of my recovery something strange happened. I was back in the emergency room with a condition called **menorrhagia**, which is bleeding at a time other than during your menstrual cycle; however, I was bleeding without a uterus. You know the first question they asked me and I am so glad I was able to answer no. However, that still did not explain why I started bleeding. I was examined and my story was confirmed. There were no signs of infection, although I was running a low grade fever of 100 and advised to remain in bed and follow-up with my physician. Alas, the mystery still remains a mystery and it was attributed to stress! Husbands, let your wives recover in peace.

Gyn Problem Visit Encounter Report
Encounter Date: 09/30/2003

Provider: M.D.   Patient: BROWN, STACEY P. (107528)

Practice: C. - Riverdale   D.O.B: 05/23/1959

Allergies: None   Current Meds: I

9/30/2003 18:38:22 Dr.   Results of TVUS/SIS explained in detail several times. Questions were encoraged and answered

CC

Gyn-Evaluation, pt is here for ultrasound.
Annual Questions   y 15:39)
    First Day of Last Menstrual Period (LMP)   Date=09/07/2003
    Smoker?   No
    List of Current Medications   #1=See mediction list; #2=

OBJECTIVE:

   15:37

     VITALS   Blood pressure: 110 mmHg/60 mmHg

LABS / X-RAYS:

   Saline Infusion Sonogram
      Cervix Nabothian cyst
      Collected
      Endometrial Lesion, Fibroid
      Endometrial Thickness=8 mm
      Intramural fibroids
      largest fibroid=8.300
      Left Ovary A-P diam.=2.8 cm (all metric)
      Left Ovary Long=3.7 cm (all metric)
      Left Ovary Transverse=2.2 cm (all metric)
      No fluid in cul de sac
      Peduncualted Fibroids
      RESULTS IN CHART
      Right Ovary A-P diam.=2.7 cm (all metric)
      Right Ovary LOng.=3.8 cm (all metric)
      Right Ovary Transverse=2.400
      Uterus A-P diam=9.1 cm (all metric)
      Uterus Long.=9.2 cm (all metric)
      Uterus Transverse=10.6 cm (all metric)

ASSESSMENT: (09/30/2003) Abnormal Laboratory Result (NOS) <796.4>

PLAN:
   Activity: <NEW> pt informed of decreased WBC's

ASSESSMENT: (09/30/2003) Menorrhagia <626.2>

PLAN:
   :   <NEW> Saline Infusion Sonogram (COMPLETED)
   Medication: <NEW> Doxycycline, Tabs 100 mg: 1 Tablet po BID x 10 Days - Rx: 20 Tablets, No refill
   Activity: <NEW> again pamphlets given
              <NEW> Again disc'd options: observation   , 2nd opinion
              <NEW> Pt will call back w/ decision

Provider: M.D.   Patient: BROWN, STACY P. (107528)
Practice: - Riverdale   D.O.B: 05/23/1959

Riverdale, GA 302/4

LABS / X-RAYS:

Hemoglobin:
    (g/dl)=1
    Collected

Wet smear
    Collected

PAP sr
  Cervix: negative for intraepithelial lesion or malignancy

Mammogram (Collected by   14:56)
  RESULTS PENDING

Transvaginal U/S   .D.
  Cervix, Nabothian cyst
  Collected
  Endometrial Stripe (mm)=8
  largest fibroid==3.8 cm (all metric)
  Left Ovary Length=3.7 cm (all metric)
  Left Ovary Width=2.1 cm (all metric)
  Myometrium, fibroids
  No or Minimal Fluid in Cul-De-Sac
  Right Ovary Length=3.1 cm (all metric)
  Right Ovary Width=1.6 cm (all metric)
  Uterine Depth=9.9 cm (all metric)
  Uterine height=10 cm (all metric)
  Uterine Width=8.4 cm (all metric)

ASSESSMENT: (12/05/2002) Leiomyoma, uterus (Unspecified) <218.0>

PLAN:
Activity: <NEW> Continue observation

ASSESSMENT: (12/05/2002) Pelvic pain <625.9>
PLAN:
:

ASSESSMEN
PLAN:
:
Medication:

Activity:

Follow Up:

ASSESSMENT
PLAN:
:   <NEW> Mammogram (COLLECTED)
     <NEW> PAP smear
Activity: <NEW>   commended

As you can see from my reports, I have every fibroid listed on this diagram. I even have one that is not listed: a myometrium fibroid. A myometrium fibroid is one located in the uterine lining and grows in the middle layer of the uterine wall. As you can imagine it is very painful. Prostaglandins act on masts cells of the uterus.

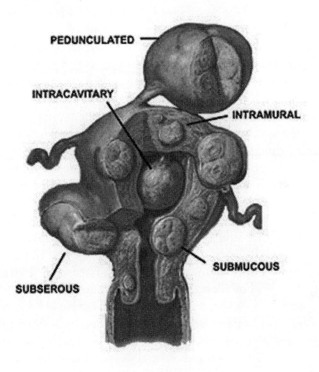

CHAPTER THIRTY

Shingles

One Saturday evening, on or about August 6, 2005, my family and I were all piled in bed watching a movie. I had been dozing off as usual, when suddenly I felt this stabbing pain on the left side of my chest. I sat up out of my sleep. I had no idea what was wrong, but I could feel this tingling sensation beneath my breast. I rushed to the bathroom holding my side. I had this unusual sensation beneath my breast. I lifted my gown and looked in the mirror. There were two pustules. One had opened and was oozing fluid. I had noticed one bump a few days earlier, but I just dismissed it as a pimple or a mosquito bite because I wear midriff blouses. I thought if I gave it time it would go away. Now that one "pimple" had sprouted into two, I looked at the reflection in horror. Somehow, deep down inside, I knew what it was shingles. I sank to the floor in disbelief. I was beside myself. How does this keep happening to me? I put a Band-Aid over it, but that only seemed to aggravate it even more. It was then that I noticed there was silence coming from the other side of the door. My family members began to call to me gently, "Are you all right?" I reassured them that I was all right through my stifled sobs because I didn't want to worry them, but I knew I wasn't all right. I was far from all right. The silence continued. I'm sure they could hear me crying because the question was repeated, and the silence continued. I knew I had to do something. So I quickly composed myself for the sake of my children. I got back into bed, reassured everyone that I was all right without saying what I thought was wrong. I got back into bed and feigned sleep. I was at the doctor's office first thing Monday morning.

The tingling and pain continued throughout the weekend, and just waiting one day felt like an eternity. By Monday I was anxious. I arrived at the doctor's office, and by then the lesions were spreading to the left across the chest wall. He confirmed what I already knew: a positive diagnosis of shingles.

Shingles is caused by a particular type of herpes virus *Varicella zoster*. There are, in fact, two types of herpes infections: genital herpes or cold sores, which are caused by the herpes simplex virus, and *Varicella zoster*. Although genital

170

herpes and cold sores come from the same virus, they are distinguished by health professionals as HSV Type 1, which refers to cold sores, and HSV Type 2, which refers to genital herpes. Interestingly enough, you can become infected with genital herpes from your partner having a cold sore or fever blister and by engaging in oral sex and vice versa. Education is everything. *Varicella zoster* causes only chicken pox and shingles. Shingles comes from a Latin word meaning "belt," and *zoster* is the Greek word for "belt." The first sign of shingles is tingling or itchiness of the skin up to one week before the rash occurs. Some people experience stabbing pains at the beginning, but others have pain only after the rash begins. The rash

Shingles

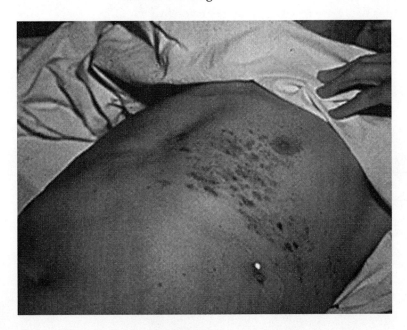

begins as a "belt" of raised dots moving to one side of the body. It may affect the face, truck, arms, legs, or abdomen. The most common site, however, is on one side of the chest and on one side of the forehead or scalp. If the lesions appear on the forehead or scalp, immediate attention is required within two to three days of the rash because it will cause blindness. Once the bumps appear, they fill up with fluid and become blisters after only a few days. It takes up to two weeks for the blisters to heal—that is, dry out, crust, and drop off. While they are in this stage, the virus is still present in the fluid located in the blister. It takes about a month for shingles to clear up, but a patient may experience pain in the blister site for years. This is called PHN, or postherpetic neuralgia. Shingles typically affects people sixty-five and older, but, as you can see in my case, there are exceptions to every rule. If you had chicken pox as a child, the virus remains dormant in your system in the nerve root cells of your body. The awakening of this virus within the nervous system is called shingles. Shingles causes a blistering rash, severe burning pain, tingling, or extreme sensitivity to the skin. The rash is usually limited to one side of the body and lasts for about one month. As such, shingles theoretically is a second outbreak of chicken pox.

Although shingles is not contagious, if you have not had chicken pox you can activate the virus in someone who had not been immunized. Statistically, one out of ten people who have had chicken pox as a child will get shingles in their lives after they have reached the age of sixty-five.

CHAPTER THIRTY-ONE

DNA/RNA

We often wonder how one person may get a disease while the other may not, or perhaps why children in the same family born from the same two parents and one of the children seems not to look like the others. The explanation for this is DNA, or deoxyribonucleic acid. Humans have twenty-three (23) pairs of chromosomes for a total of forty six (46). Each parent contributes twenty-three. These DNA strands are randomly chosen. When the egg is fertilized by the male sperm, the two strands contained in each combine to form a single strand. In order to form a single strand, characteristics from each are randomly chosen as copies from each gene from either parent are passed directly to the child. Because gene selection is so random, each child will get a different mix of genes from the DNA of the same mother and father. That is why children from the same parents can have so many differences.

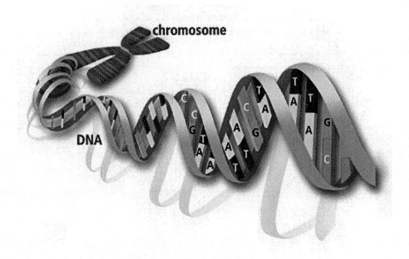

A mutant or recessive gene is one that can be carried through many generations and never be noticed until, at some point, both parents contribute a copy of that mutant or recessive gene. Some children are born with ethnic-specific diseases such as sickle cell anemia, which is likely to occur among African Americans, or Tay-Sachs disease, which is common among people of Jewish, French Canadian, or Mediterranean ancestry. This happens when there is a small gene pool, and it limits variation. As such genetic problems, deformities and fertility problems occur. A large gene pool provides a genetic buffer against genetic diseases, and the probability that genetic diseases will be passed on. The wider the gene pool, the lesser the chance that the offspring will have problems. However, through my personal journey, I have learned what my aunt Elizabeth meant by what she had been telling me all my life, that blood will tell. Although they may lie dormant, when you have been diagnosed with a rare disease and you are outside of a so-called statistical group, the likelihood is gene mutation or a recessive gene. A gene mutation occurs in two ways: it can be inherited or acquired. An inherited mutation is present in every cell in that person's body. DNA actually dates back approximately 3.5 to 4.6 billions of years. DNA is responsible for everything, from your hair color and texture to your eye color. For African Americans, most of us are unaware of our mixed ancestral traits unless you have traced them back, like Alex Haley did in *Roots* or *Oprah*. What a wonderful discovery it must be to know your complete family history and to actually meet your family members from other countries such as Africa, Ireland, Japan, England, etc. On the other hand, an acquired mutation can occur in the DNA of an individual cell at some time during that person's life, caused by environmental factors such as ultraviolet radiation from the sun, to your grandfather having been exposed to chemicals at his job before you were conceived. Acquired mutation cannot be copied and passed on to the next generation; however, mutated cells have been linked to cancer. However, if an inherited mutation occurs during a person's life, there is a chance that the mutation will be passed on to that person's children.

DNA is a pair of molecules joined together by hydrogen bonds. There is no such thing as a single molecule, because they all come in pairs organized in two complementary strands. These two strands contain combined genetic information deoxyribozyme or DNA enzyme. It is an instruction manual for the body, and it makes copies of itself.

RNA is single stranded. Its job is to translate DNA messages into proteins. Just like the game telephone, those messages can be flawed, and the body has no way to detect or repair those flaws. The transfer RNA is what carries the instructions of messages to the cells, and they operate ten times faster than DNA. The message centers of the RNA are called ribosomes. These message centers are located throughout the cell, and they translate the chains of amino acids.

An organ and cell are composed of proteins, and their job is to chemically break down food in order to fight disease.

An autoimmune disease occurs when the body attacks itself, and there is no cure. The body has produced an immune response against its own tissues. In certain types of autoimmune diseases, a bacteria or virus triggers an immune response, and the antibodies or the T cells attack the normal cells. As such, the body attacks itself, thinking it is attacking an infecting germ. Such is the case with multiple sclerosis. There are two general categories of autoimmune diseases: systemic and localized. Systemic autoimmune diseases are those that damage many organs such as lupus or rheumatoid arthritis. When only a single organ or tissue is damaged, such as the central nervous system in multiple sclerosis, then this is referred to as a localized autoimmune disease. Although the central nervous system controls the whole body, it is considered a single system.

Beyond the function of replicating life, DNA is a nucleic acid and contains genetic instructions for biological development of a cellular form of life or a virus. Everything has a genetic code and is susceptible to it, especially diseases. With that in mind, we have to understand how it works. Red blood cells carry oxygen throughout the body. DNA contains messenger functions, including the transport of hormones and the signaling of tissue damage, immunological functions, including the circulation of white cells and detection of foreign material by antibodies, regulation of core body temperature, removal of waste, etc. Viruses contain genetic material. Mutations are changes to genetic material caused by copying errors during cell division and by exposure to radiation, chemicals, or viruses; and this is passed on to descendants. Most of your DNA is located in the cell nucleus. We assume that DNA gene coding has finished its work at the time of your birth, but that is merely an assumption. Inside a gene, there remains a part called an **exon**, or an open reading frame. This part of the gene is waiting to complete instructions in the body for things such as diseases or viruses. The term *exon* was coined in 1978 by Walter Gilbert. Before the instructions become RNA, they go through a rigorous process.

The doubling of DNA is called replication. In the process of replication, however, the body may attempt to correct or repair an abnormality, and cancer may develop in the offspring. This is why cell division and generational information is so important. RNA transcription occurs when it translates or in effect follows the instructions mapped out by the genes or DNA. In order to maintain life, DNA has to stay intact so RNA works like a reference book of the DNA on a short-term basis and translates the available information. When a gene is copied, then it must undergo a three-step process before it can leave the cell and be translated into protein for use by the body. The first process is called **capping**. A special nucleotide is attached to the end of the RNA in order to stabilize it. This process is necessary to ensure efficient initiation of protein synthesis. The second part of the process involves a special enzyme **attaching** a chain of 150 to 200 adenine nucleotides to the three-inch end of the pre-mRNA directly after transcription. This process increases stability and prolongs the life of the mRNA molecule. The final process is called **splicing**. It involves the removal of noncoding sequences from pre-mRNA in order to create mRNA. The result will contain only the coding sequences for a protein—a special complex called a splicosome, consisting of proteins and catalytic nuclear RNA molecules, snRNAs. (Exon is an open frame, and an Intron is an unused gene frame.) The next process is called **transport**. DNA is transcribed into mRNA in the nucleus; protein synthesis takes place in the cytoplasm, and then the mRNA has to exit the nucleus to the cytoplasm. Since the nucleus and the cytoplasm are completely two separate environments, they are enclosed by a double membrane and connected to each other through what is called a nuclear pore complex. When it is time for the mRNA to leave the nucleus and enter the cytoplasm, it is "tagged" by proteins, which direct the mRNA to leave its environment. It then attaches to export receptors, and export proteins are translocated through the nuclear pore complex. The mRNA is now ready for the final step. It is ready to be released into the cytoplasm and RNA translation. Your muscles, hair, eyes, etc., are all made of protein. Proteins are the building blocks of life.

RNA has its own language. The information contained in a nucleotide sequence of mRNA is read as three-letter words called condons or triplets. Each word represents an amino acid, and during translation, the acids are linked together to form a polypeptide chain. This chain is later folded into a protein, and translation is dependent upon several components: initiation, elongation, and termination. The translation process begins when ribosome charged with tRNA and amino acid methionine encounters mRNA. The ribosome will attach and begin to scan the mRNA and look for a start signal. When the start sequence is found, this is AUG, the condon (triplet) for amino acid methionine. The large subunit will join the small subunit and form a complete ribosome; the complete protein synthesis is initiated.

The next step is **elongation**. As a result of initiation, a new tRNA and amino acid has entered the ribosome. The anticondon will move downstream of the AUG condon, and if it matches the mRNA, then the basepairs and the ribosome can link the two amino acids together. If there is no match, then it will be rejected. The ribosome moves one triplet forward, and the process is repeated.

The final step is **termination**. After the process repeats and the ribosome has reached one of three stop condons, then termination proteins will bind to the ribosome and stimulate release of the polypeptide chain (protein) and then the ribosome will disassociate from the mRNA. When disassociation occurs, translation begins again. Some cells need larger quantities of a protein and, as such, translation and modification may take longer before the RNA becomes fully active.

The genetic code contains four basic alternating sequences: adenine (A), guanine (G), cytosine (C), and uracil (U). Each alternating sequence consists of twenty amino acids naturally found in protein. It was discovered in 1960 that one condon represents twenty amino acids, and each condon is represented by a letter. The genetic code has no commas and can be written like a language and translated by following nucleotides three at a time. There is no particular start point. It was also discovered that by following these principles, there were sixty-four possible combinations. In 1968, Nirenberg and Khorana won the Nobel Prize in Physiology and Medicine for discovering the genetic code.

The biological function of the human body can be interrupted by outside forces, causing damage to the DNA. The result will be disease, organ dysfunction, and, as we have seen here, even death. Damage to the DNA strand is referred to as mutagens. A mutagen is where a physical or chemical agent changes the genetic information (DNA), causing a mutation in that organism. The mutation can occur deliberately, causing changes to the base pair sequence of the genetic material of an organism. When Vioxx was introduced into the bloodstream of a patient, it immediately changed the DNA of the individual causing changes to the genetic material. Remember the sixth receptor, gap junction, cardiac disturbance? This is why there were a record number of heart attacks, strokes, and medical injuries reported due to ingesting Vioxx, Bextra, and Celebrex. When there was subsequent DNA mutation, the gap junctions will not repeat as they were genetically programmed to do.

CHAPTER THIRTY-TWO

Prescription Drugs/Informed Consent

I was cleaning my home one morning and had the television on for company when I looked up and saw a commercial. "SUICIDE, SUICIDE, SUICIDE." I turned off the vacuum cleaner to listen. It was a legal advertisement to join a class action lawsuit for prescription medication. It seems that several antidepressant medications had proven adverse side effects and had caused individuals to commit suicide or attempt suicide. Then I saw the list of drugs roll on the television screen. I heard the announcer, but it was in absolute disbelief because it did not register the first time. I sat there and waited for the commercial to air again. Within the hour, there it was again. When I saw the list for the second time, I couldn't close my mouth. The drugs were listed as antidepressants. I said to myself, "I'm not taking an antidepressant. My doctor wouldn't do this to me." The drug prescribed was Neurontin. It was prescribed the first time for PHN, post-herpetic neuralgia, the pain experienced after shingles, and the second time for an exacerbation of multiple sclerosis—burning in the legs. After the shock wore off, I got angry. You know the old saying, "Hindsight is twenty-twenty." I started to think back to when I started taking the drug. It all started to make sense. I complained of excessive urination. The doctor responded with a round of steroids and explained it was a side effect and that I was having another exacerbation of multiple sclerosis. I refused the steroids because there was no evidence of urinary tract infection. I realize that I am a doctor's worst nightmare. I question everything, but obviously I didn't ask enough questions. We all have personal problems, and some have more than most. I have my faith in God, and I stand on that, as such I adamantly refused to take antidepressants. My doctor should have respected my position, which I made clear on more than one occasion. Murphy's law seems to have been fully operational between 2000 and 2006. I lost two brothers and a cousin, one from cancer and two in freak automobile accidents. I was diagnosed with several illnesses. I woke up at 6:00 a.m. and caught some men stealing speakers out of my car in my driveway at gunpoint. My sister had just been told she was misdiagnosed, not a fibroid, but a tumors attached to the ovaries. I was having marital trouble and financial trouble.

The kids were going through growing pains. Mom was sick and hospitalized. You name it, I was going through it. I asked myself what else could go wrong. I couldn't figure out why all these bad things wouldn't stop happening. Then to make matters worse, I couldn't get a handle my health, and I was having another multiple sclerosis exacerbation. Have mercy, Jesus! It is a natural human response to cry. That is why God put tear ducts in our eyes and gave us that ability. That's why they are called emotions. When we are overwhelmed, we pray. When we have a problem, we try and find solutions, and we solve them. As far as I am concerned, you don't take a pill for a problem that needs to be worked out, talked out, or financially relieved. If you cannot change it, then we have to learn to accept it or adapt or change our circumstances. Period! As King Solomon said, "There is nothing new under the sun. We only reinvent ways to solve old problems."

Dr. Grace Jackson revealed in her book, *Rethinking Psychiatric Drugs: A Guide to Informed Consent*, that 20 percent of Americans **unknowingly** take these drugs and consume them on a regular basis. These drugs stress the brain, and they do more harm than good. There is an obvious crisis in medical ethics, and there is a responsibility to patients. I obviously had a right to refuse consent to take that drug, and that consent was taken away from me. My family noticed the obvious change in my behavior; my church members thought a twig snapped. I have trust issues now with health professionals after my personal experiences.

Neurontin was also prescribed to women undergoing menopause. The drug alleviated hot flashes; however, the drug was also prescribed to patients who failed to respond to antidepressants or mood stabilizers. The drug was successful in the treatment of those with mixed bipolar states and antipsychotic induced tardive dyskinesia. Tardive dyskinesia is a drug-induced neurological disease that is irreversible. Neurontin was successful in treating this serious disease. Those patients who had been chemically lobotomized with neuroleptic drugs such as Haldol, Thorazine, and lithium now suffering tardive dyskinesia were treated with Neurontin and remarkably showed improvement where otherwise the disease was thought to have been untreatable. Those who marketed Neurontin were aware of its side effects, which included the psychiatric reactions of mania, paranoia, sexual side effects, and suicidal thoughts. But they approved the drug anyway, because of the "other" benefits, because the drug proved *so* promising. It was also proven that the drug stopped nerve pain in postherpetic neuralgia, and it was useful in diseases associated with diabetes and neuropathic pain such as multiple sclerosis.

The only problem associated with those taking Neurontin is that they, like me, were unaware of its antidepressant side effects and its effect on the brain, until now. When a significant number of citizens attempt or commit suicide, as an outcome of the side effects of the drug, then we pay attention. Just being armed with this information is enough to make you want to raise the roof, but the question is, who is to be held accountable? The damage was already done. Dr.

Peter Breggin penned over nineteen books and articles about the dangers, that these drugs actually do more harm than good. Dr. Breggin is a criminal psychiatrist and has been in private practice since 1968. He advised that withdrawal can be worse than actually taking the drugs, and the effects may last a lifetime, although it took your doctor fifteen minutes to write the prescription. Dr. Breggin found that the effects are emotional, physical, and life-long if not taken under doctor's supervision. **If you were not a psychiatric patient to begin with, there will obviously be effects on the brain.** This fact is what concerned me the most.

Our elderly are tossed aside like rotten garbage into nursing homes and administered chemical straightjackets to keep them from moving from their beds or wheelchairs and to keep them from complaining. Eventually they become another casualty of tardive dyskinesia. Well, who's listening if they can't complain? These drugs are being administered against their will; chemical rape, if you will. Antidepressants disrupt normal brain function and cause long-term damage.

The public has long been under the impression that depression is caused by an imbalance in the brain—a dysfunction of a neurotransmitter called serotonin. Pharmaceutical companies and psychiatrists have long held that pills are the answer to the problem. Scientists tried everything from increasing levels of serotonin to lowering levels, yet years of varieties of drug therapy resulted in suicide and homicidal behavior. A man with no prior criminal history and no former social pattern of violence found himself facing a rape charge. Dr. Peter Breggin testified in the postconviction hearing that the antidepressants caused the young man to engage in sexually deviant behavior and this, in fact, contributed to his crime. He proved that the manufacturer was aware of the side effects of these drugs before they were prescribed and that this individual was just a casualty of their side effects. Initially, the judge was skeptical; however, after reviewing the overwhelming evidence and reports as to the drug-induced side effects, instead of sentencing this young man to two consecutive life sentences with no parole, he was given twenty-one years with release in nineteen years. (Charleston County Court, November 15, 2001, Andrew Savage, Esq. Attorney for the defendant, Dr. Peter Breggin, Medical Expert for the defense, Judge Edward Cottinham.) There are many cases of involuntary intoxication and "**acting out**" caused by these antidepressants. There were other cases of "acting out" that included malicious wounding, kidnapping, etc.—all of them adverse drug reactions. The bottom line here is whether an antidepressant is ingested voluntarily or involuntarily.

Depression cannot be cured with medication. It is only a Band-Aid. In the Holy Bible, God said in Genesis 1:29, "Behold, I have given you every herb-bearing seed which is upon the face of the earth, and every tree, in which is the fruit of a tree yielding seed; to you it shall be for meat." God made these bodies and knows what's best. History and study have proven that when there is an imbalance in the body, then illness will result. Shouldn't the same rules apply to emotional illness?

The Archives of General Psychiatry reported in 2002 that a gram of fish oil a day decreased symptoms of anxiety, sleep disorders, feelings of sadness, depression, suicidal thoughts, and decreased sex drive. Raw vegetables, especially cabbage, whole grains, seeds, nuts are all good for the brain and have been proven to boost brain function. We have all heard on the news that refined sugar, caffeine, smoking, lack of exercise all lead to depression and should be avoided. You are your best advocate. Ask questions, and if you are not satisfied, ask again.

As previously indicated, when there is an imbalance, the body will not properly function—and that includes emotional as well as physical. Doctors have known that vitamin deficiency can also cause depression. Absent social factors, a diet lacking in niacin and tryptophan will result in depression. But who is going to test for niacin and tryptophan (an amino acid produced in the digestive process) deficiency? Obvious signs of this imbalance are weight loss, glossitis of the tongue (abnormality of the tongue resulting from inflammation), dermatitis, weight loss, diarrhea, depression, and dementia. B6 deficiency has been linked to attention-deficit disorder. B12 has been linked to memory loss, hallucinations, disorientation, and dementia.

It was revealed during discovery at trial that when Vioxx hit the market in 1999, the company conducted clinical trials. They used Vioxx at 25-milligram doses and dummy tablets. The study was conducted over a three-year period, and the purpose of the study was to prevent polyps of the colon and rectum. The trial was stopped after the drug company discovered that those not taking the dummy pills experienced a 50 percent incidence of heart attack and sudden cardiac death compared to the other group. Even after this group study, they went on to spend $160.8 million in a television marketing campaign, featuring figure skater Dorothy Hamill to advertise the drug without telling her that by ingesting the drug, there will be risk of heart attack four times greater on Vioxx. When a health advocacy group in Washington DC found out the truth about Vioxx in 2000, Sid Wolfe, a physician and director of the health research group of the advocacy group Public Citizen of Washington DC, said, "Dorothy Hamill doesn't tell people they have four times the risk of heart attack on Vioxx."

I was one of the first patients to take it. I took it without question. Why do most of us take medication? Because we trust our doctors, and we trust their judgment. The doctors take a Hippocratic oath, and the pharmacist takes a pharmaceutical oath, but who is watching the pharmaceutical companies? I am not diminishing their contributions to our society, but just like professional lobbyists they wine and dine our doctors into using their samples and new products hot off the shelves. Without question they are prescribed to people like me who are suffering, and, as I indicated, I would have taken anything to have relieved my symptoms. However, was it informed consent? I was opting for relief from burning. I go to church to relieve myself from the pressures of the world and to praise

God, and he did not have the right to make that decision for me. According to the July 1, 1999, United States population census, the population was 273,000 million, and 1.9 percent represents approximately 2.6 million people. When the drug company finished running their trials in 1999 and completed their results, they knew that, give or take, these are the number of people that would potentially be sick, injured, or killed as a result of taking the drug if it were released on the market. Again that's **approximately 2.6 million people representing 1.9 percent in a class possibly affected.** Out of that number, these were the potential litigants, and the drug company felt it was safe to proceed to market anyway.

Clinical data at trial revealed that the drug company conducted a three-year study using 25 milligram doses of Vioxx. And when Vioxx, Bextra, and Celebrex hit the market, the pharmaceutical company knew that, statistically, only 0.1 percent to 1.9 percent treated with Vioxx, Bextra, or Celebrexx would potentially suffer any of the following side effects:

Body as a whole: abdominal distension, abdominal tenderness, abscess, chest pain, chills, contusion, cyst, diaphragmatic hernia, fever, fluid retention, flushing, fungal infection, infection pain, laceration, pelvic pain, peripheral edema, postoperative pain, syncope, trauma, upper extremity edema, viral syndrome, hematuria.

Cardiovascular System: angina pectoris, atrial fibrillation, bradycardia, irregular heartbeat, palpitation, hematoma, premature ventricular contraction, tachycardia, venous insufficiency.

Digestive System: acid reflux, aphthous stomatitis, dental caries, dental pain, digestive gas symptoms, dry mouth, duodenal disorder (intestinal), dysgeusia, esophagitis, flatulence, gastric disorder, gastritis, gastroenteritis and infectious gastroenteritis, hematochezia, hemorrhoids, oral infection, oral ulcer, oral lesion, vomiting.

Eyes, Ears, Nose, and Throat: allergic rhinitis, blurred vision, cerumen impaction, conjunctivitis, dry throat, epistaxis, laryngitis, nasal congestion and secretion, ophthalmic injection, optic pain, otitis, otitis media, pharyngitis, tinnitus, tonsillitis.

Immune System: allergy, hypersensitivity, insect bite reaction, leukopenia, anemia, lymphoma, Steven Johnson's syndrome.

Metabolism and Nutrition: appetite change, hypercholesterolemia, weight gain.

Musculoskeletal: ankle sprain, arm pain, arthralgia, back strain, bursitis, cartilage trauma, joint swelling, muscular cramp, muscular disorder, muscular weakness, musculoskeletal pain and stiffness, myalgia, osteoarthritis, tendonitis, traumatic arthropathy, wrist fracture.

Nervous System: hyperesthesia, insomnia, median nerve neuropathy, migraine, muscular spasm, paresthesia, sciatica, somnolence (drowsiness), vertigo.

Emotional: anxiety, depression, mental acuity decreased.

Respiratory System: asthma, cough, dyspnea, pneumonia, pulmonary congestion, respiratory infection, abrasion, alopecia, atopic dermatitis, basal cell carcinoma, blister, cellulitis, contact dermatitis, herpes simplex and zoster, nail unit disorder, perspiration, pruritus (severe itching of undamaged skin), rash, skin erythema, urticaria, xerosis.

Urogenital System: breast mass, cystitis, dysuria, menopausal symptoms, menstrual disorder, nocturia, urinary retention, vaginitis.

As I indicated, the pharmaceutical industry is a multibillion-dollar industry. Justice finally came on November 9, 2007, but the litigants have yet to receive their just reward. I provided you with proof of all the disorders I acquired after taking Vioxx and Celebrex. Do you think this is a coincidence? Most of the diagnoses came back to back. They are permanent. Based on the aforementioned information, I ask you to make an informed decision. I became one of the 1.9 percent. Who is to be held accountable? I am the one who has to live with the outcome of their statistical data. But I am not a piece of paper. I'm living, breathing, and suffering on a daily basis; and there is no cure for these diseases. You've read my radiology reports and blood tests. They don't lie.

I am reminded that it could have been worse, God didn't have to wake me up this morning. I have a home, I have my family. And no matter how bad you think your situation is, there is always someone out there worse off than you are. God spared me to allow me to tell my story.

I am silver in my Father's hands. "He will sit as a refiner and purifier of silver" (Malachi 3:3). As a silversmith holds silver over the fire, such is my life. A silversmith holds the silver over the fire and burns away all the impurities so that the silver can be refined. As he holds the silver, he cannot take his eyes away from the silver or leave it in the fire too long or else it will be destroyed. The silversmith knows that the silver is ready—when he sees his image in the silver!

PICTURE FILE

35. Image 35.   Nabothian: www.emedicine.net
36. Image 36.   Fibroid: *www.uefinfo.com*
37. Image 37.   Shingles: virology-online.com
38. Image 38.   DNA Helix: wwwscotfamily.com
39. Image 39:   Sciatica: *www.chiropracticchicagohousecalls.com*
40. Image 42   Eye: academia.hixie.ch
41. Image 68   Lymphatic System: www.phoenix5.org